A CONSUMER'S GUIDE TO CONTACT LENSES

A CONSUMER'S GUIDE TO CONTACT LENSES

BY

SPENCER E. SHERMAN

M.D., F.A.C.S.
Diplomate, American Board of Ophthalmology

WITH

NANCY P. BRUNING

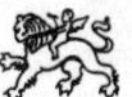

THE DIAL PRESS
New York

Published by
The Dial Press
1 Dag Hammarskjold Plaza
New York, New York 10017

Manufactured in the United States of America

First printing

Design by Elaine Golt Gongora

Drawings by Robert Frank

Library of Congress Cataloging in Publication Data

Sherman, Spencer E.
A consumer's guide to contact lenses.

Bibliography: p.
Includes index.
1. Contact lenses. 2. Consumer education.
I. Bruning, Nancy. II. Title.
RE977.C6S46 617.7'523 81-19464
ISBN 0-385-27403-3 AACR2

ACKNOWLEDGMENTS

The authors would like to thank the representatives of the following manufacturers of contact lenses and accessories for providing background material that proved invaluable to our research: Alcon Optic; American Hydron; Amsco Lombart Lenses; Barnes-Hind Pharmaceuticals, Inc.; Bausch & Lomb; Blairex Laboratories; Ciba Vision Care; Cooper Vision; Danker Laboratories, Inc.; Dow Corning Ophthalmics; Heyer-Schulte Medical Optics Center; Hydrocurve Soft Lenses, Inc.; Medicornea; Milton Roy Company; Neefe Optical Laboratory; Salvatori Ophthalmics, Inc.; Syntex Ophthalmics, Inc.; and Wesley-Jessen, Inc. We would also like to acknowledge the assistance of the Contact Lens Manufacturers Association and the Food and Drug Administration Division of Ophthalmic, Ear, Nose, Throat, and Dental Devices. Finally, our thanks and appreciation to Robert Frank, whose fine drawings illustrate our text so well.

I dedicate
this book to
Susan,
Sabrina,
and Cristine
for all their
love and support

TABLE OF CONTENTS

PREFACE

About one out of two Americans—that's 115 million people—are unable to see with the naked eye alone. More and more are refusing to be burdened with spectacles and are opting for the modern form of vision correction: contact lenses. It has been estimated there are between eleven and fourteen million contact lens wearers, and that one and a half million newcomers join these ranks every year. In response to this growing demand contact lens technology and manufacture are booming: there are dozens and dozens of manufacturers and brands, and places to buy contact lenses are cropping up like mushrooms. This has created a broad range of choices, which is good. Unfortunately the widespread availability of contact lenses has also created a great deal of confusion and misinformation in the mind of the past, present, and future contact lens wearer. Of the annual one and a half million new contact lens wearers an astounding 30 to 40 percent drop out during the first twelve to twenty-four months; obviously some more fall by the wayside after that. This failure rate suggests a lot of misspent time and money, contact lenses sitting in dresser drawers, and a great number of frustrated people walking around. This doesn't have to be. It is my belief that a well-informed consumer has the best chance of wearing contact lenses successfully. Thus, *A Consumer's Guide to Contact Lenses* was written to answer the questions, to fill in the gaps, to allay the fears, and to dispel the myths that cloud this interesting subject.

For example:

Do people see better with contact lenses than with glasses?
Yes, usually (see p. 16).

How do you know whether you can really wear contact lenses; or whether you should wear hard, soft, gas-permeable, or extended-wear lenses?
The answers to these questions can only be determined by an expert in the contact lens field: an ophthalmologist or optometrist who specializes in contact lenses (see pp. 20–21).

Why can't someone go to a "bargain center" and get a pair of lenses or a replacement lens?
The old adage that you get what you pay for is especially true here (see pp. 22–24).

Do contact lenses prevent the eyes from becoming worse?
No (see p. 166).

Can the eyes become dependent on contact lenses?
No (see p. 160).

Can a contact lens become lost behind the eye?
No (see p. 170).

Is it true that wearing contact lenses for many years can damage the eyes?
Sometimes; but for more than 99 percent of the contact lens wearers no damage to the eye ever occurs (see p. 162).

Is it permissible to clean a contact lens by putting it in your mouth?
Absolutely not (see p. 161).

A Consumer's Guide to Contact Lenses gives detailed answers to all these questions—and many more. In the following chapters you'll find out how your eyes work; learn about different types of lenses (including the new extended-wear lenses that stay in your eyes during sleep and comfortable soft lenses that correct astigmatism); how to handle, wear, and care for them; and where to go to obtain the right contact lenses for you. I also discuss how to take care of any problems with contact lenses that might crop up, and explode a few myths about contact lenses that might have kept you from considering them.

The perfect contact lens has yet to be developed. But technological advances are constantly bringing us closer to the moment when contact lenses will provide perfect vision—and will be able to be worn constantly and comfortably. Until that happy day *A Consumer's Guide to Contact Lenses* will help you to approach perfect sight with your lenses and to join the legions of satisfied contact lens wearers discussed in this book. Today the chances are very good indeed that you will be able to wear contact lenses—and this is true even if you've tried in the past and were unsuccessful. It's important, though, to realize that while contact lens wear seems simple—you just pop them in and pop them out—there's far more to contact lenses than meets the eye.

CHAPTER ONE

A LOOK AT CONTACT LENSES

WHAT ARE CONTACT LENSES?

The contact lens worn today is a tiny, thin, dome-shaped, transparent disc that's usually made from special types of plastic and sometimes silicone rubber. Most hard lenses are a mere 8 to 10 mm in diameter and .035 to 1 mm thick. (One inch equals 22 mm.) Soft lenses are a bit larger, but most are 11 to 16 mm in diameter or less. Such precision and delicacy weren't always the case. How something that's smaller and thinner than your fingernail—sometimes as thin as a single human hair—can take the place of a pair of bulky eyeglasses is a wondrous story of how modern science and technology were put to use by scientists, innovators, and dreamers who stubbornly believed that a good idea can always get better.

The concept of contact lenses has actually been around for nearly five hundred years. As far as we know, the first contact lens was envisioned by the man who seemed to think of everything first: Leonardo da Vinci. His notebooks show that in 1508 he conceived the idea that a "little ampule of glass" could be placed on the eye in order to improve the wearer's vision. In 1636 Descartes published his own version of the contact lens: a tube filled with water. But the idea remained a gleam in everyone's eye until technology began to catch up with these two far-reaching thinkers.

The real history of the contact lens did not begin until the early nineteenth century, when Thomas Young described his idea of securing a lens from a small microscope to a tube of water. He placed the open end of the tube directly on his eye; the lens was at the far end. With some fine tuning, he was able to use this device (quite similar to Descartes's blueprint) to correct his own faulty vision.

Next, in 1823, Sir John F. W. Herschel, an English astronomer, made it widely known that he believed that vision could be corrected by placing a contact lens directly on the *cornea* (the transparent front surface of the eye that covers the pupil and iris). He proposed that the back surface of the lens fit the cornea exactly, and be made from a mold of the cornea. Though feasible in theory no mold could be made at that time because there was no effective local anesthesia available that could desensitize the exquisitely sensitive cornea.

Finally, in 1887, came the next giant step in the progress of contact lenses. A German glassblower created a glass disc designed to be worn by a person with a diseased eyelid. The lens would act as a clear protective bandage that prevented the lid from touching the eyeball. A year after that contact lenses that could correct faulty vision were made and tested. But only a few souls with wills of iron and a high tolerance for pain could wear these lenses for more than what must have been an excruciating hour. It's a wonder that anyone could wear them at all, as first they had to endure the rather crude fitting process—which then consisted of a trial-and-error approach: One glass lens after another was inserted until they found one that fit better than the others. A trial set of such lenses consisted of up to one thousand lenses! These lenses were large and covered not only the cornea, but the *sclera* (white of the eye) as well. They had to be large because they were made of glass. Consequently the weight of the glass contact lens and the pull of gravity made proper centering of the contact lens on the eye very difficult.

Those heavy (and dangerous) contact lenses eventually gave way to the breakthrough that marked the beginning of safe and comfortable contact lens wear. It came in the 1930s when an American optometrist, William Feinbloom, created the first plastic lenses. They were fitted by taking impressions of the wearer's eyes with a soft waxlike substance which subsequently hardened. From the resultant mold, a plastic contact lens was produced. Although these rigid contact lenses were still quite large and covered most of the sclera, they had the advantage of being lightweight and unbreakable. One of

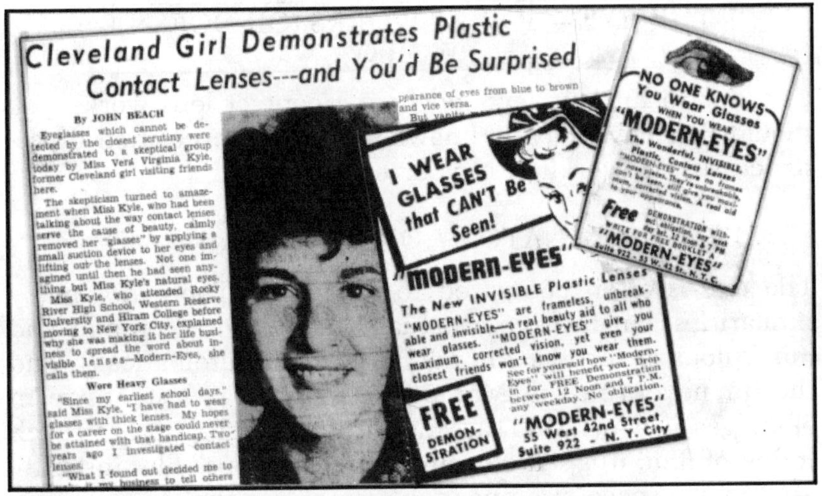

Cleveland Girl Demonstrates Plastic Contact Lenses---and You'd Be Surprised

By JOHN BEACH

Eyeglasses which cannot be detected by the closest scrutiny were demonstrated to a skeptical group today by Miss Vera Virginia Kyle, former Cleveland girl visiting friends here.

The skepticism turned to amazement when Miss Kyle, who had been talking about the way contact lenses serve the cause of beauty, calmly removed her "glasses" by applying a small suction device to her eyes and lifting out the lenses. Not one imagined until then he had seen anything but Miss Kyle's natural eyes.

Miss Kyle, who attended Rocky River High School, Western Reserve University and Hiram College before moving to New York City, explained why she was making it her life business to spread the word about invisible lenses—Modern-Eyes, she calls them.

Wore Heavy Glasses

"Since my earliest school days," said Miss Kyle, "I have had to wear glasses with thick lenses. My hopes for a career on the stage could never be attained with that handicap. Two years ago I investigated contact lenses.

"What I found out decided me to ... it my business to tell others

... pearance of eyes from blue to brown and vice versa.

But vanity ...

Figure 1. Contact lenses first became popular in the 1940s.

my patients, who was fitted with one of these original large plastic contact lenses, recounted the weeks of agony that she had to endure until her eyes adapted to the lenses. Once adapted, she could only wear the "invisible glasses" (as they were called) comfortably for a maximum of a few hours each day.

In the 1950s such scleral lenses gave way to the smaller corneal lens, which covers only the cornea. Since then hard contact lenses have gradually become smaller and thinner; now properly fitted ones can be worn all day.

The latest major innovation is, of course, the soft contact lens, which was invented in Czechoslovakia in 1960. After rigorous testing the new, revolutionary, more comfortable lens was marketed in the U.S. in 1971, making contact lenses feasible for many who were unable (or unwilling) to adapt to hard lenses.

Even more recent is the gas-permeable lens, which allows an exchange of oxygen and carbon dioxide, enabling the lenses to be worn longer and more comfortably. Soft extended-wear lenses have also been approved, allowing continuous wear for days, weeks, and even months in some cases.

THE EYE—HOW IT WORKS (OR DOESN'T WORK)

In order to fully understand how a contact lens works, you should first have a basic knowledge and appreciation of the structure and workings of your eyes.

ANATOMY OF THE EYE

The eye is often compared to a camera. There *are* many similarities, but the eye is actually much more complex and miraculous: it focuses and adjusts to light automatically, and the film never runs out. Moreover it picks up a constant stream of images, in contrast to the single image that registers on each frame of film; it is self-cleaning and "develops" film instantly —all in the space of a one-inch-diameter globe!

When you "see" something, your eyes actually pick up the light rays that are bouncing off that object. Whether you're reading a comic book, watching the ballet, or admiring a distant landscape, here's what happens: As the light rays enter your eye, they pass through and are refracted (bent) by the:

Cornea, the clear, dome-shaped tissue that covers the inner parts of the eye as a watch crystal covers the face of a watch, and which acts as the "window" of the eye. The cornea is in part responsible for focusing the light rays; unlike the crystalline lens, the shape and focusing power remain constant. The cornea, upon which the contact lens floats over a layer of tears, is the most sensitive part of the eye, since it has the highest density of nerve endings per square millimeter. Light rays then pass through the:

Pupil, the small hole that appears black at the center of the:

Iris, the blue-, green-, or brown-colored part of the eye. The pupil opens up (dilates) or closes down (constricts) automatically to adjust to the amount of light, like the shutter of a camera. The rays of light continue their journey through the:

Crystalline lens, which is clear and flexible and changes shape via muscle contraction and relaxation, depending upon the distance of the object from the eye. (This is called *accommodation.*) As the light is being focused by the lens, it passes through the:

Vitreous humor, the clear jellylike fluid that fills the inside

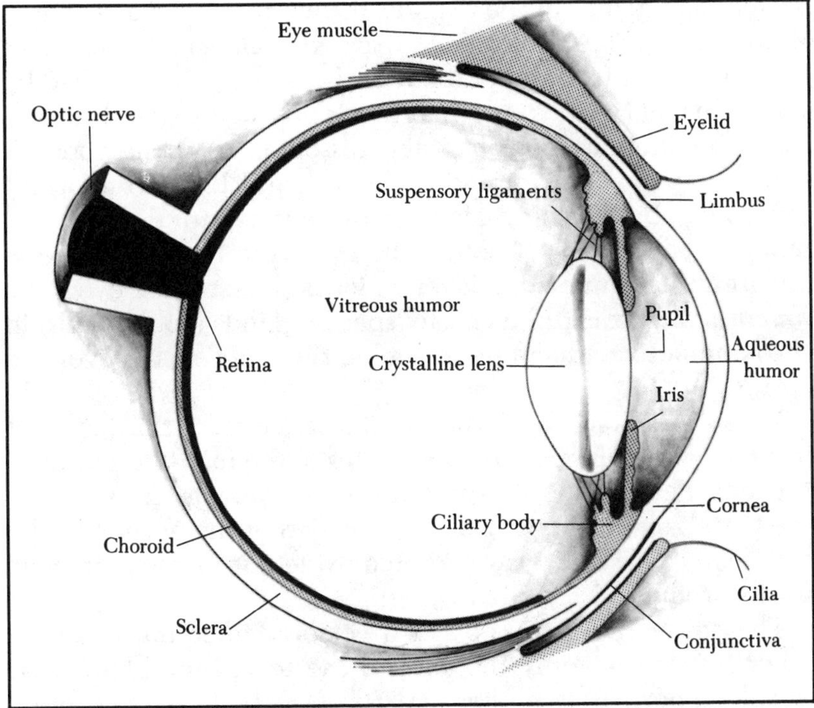

Figure 2. Anatomy of the eye.

of the eyeball and gives it its shape. It finally ends up focusing (or being out of focus, if your eye has a refractive error) on the:

Retina, or "film." This thin, delicate sheet of light-sensitive tissue lining the back of the eye is connected to the:

Optic nerve, which transmits the image in the form of a chemical-electrical impulse to the brain for decoding and interpretation.

Some parts of the eye do not relate directly to the light rays that provide the visual image, but are important for the contact lens wearer.

The conjunctiva is a thin, clear tissue that covers the white part of the eye (sclera) and undersides of the lids. This continuous sheet forms the anatomical barrier that prevents a contact lens from becoming "lost" behind the eye.

Tears play a most important part in making contact lens wear a reality. There are actually three layers to the tears. The outermost layer is *lipid,* the product of the oil-producing

Meibomian glands of the eyelids. It functions to retard evaporation of the middle layer of tears, the *aqueous layer.* This portion accounts for 40 percent of the tears. It is produced by the lachrymal glands, the main tear-producing glands of the eye. The aqueous layer contains dissolved minerals (sodium, chloride, potassium), protein, glucose, and the all-important immunoglobulins and lysozyme (the eye's natural antibodies and enzymes), which protect the eye from harmful bacteria and fungi. The innermost layer which is closest to the eye is the *mucin layer.* It is produced by special glands (goblet cells) in the conjunctiva. Mucin helps spread the tears evenly over the cornea.

When a contact lens is worn, it floats over a thin layer of tears, which cushions and contributes to the focusing power of the lens. Perhaps most important to the contact lens wearer is the tears' role in carrying a large portion of the oxygen to the cornea and carrying away carbon dioxide, the prime metabolic waste product.

The cornea itself has no blood vessels and so must rely on other sources—mainly the air and the tears—to obtain what the blood normally supplies to parts of the body. Since contact lenses diminish the amount of air reaching the cornea, the tears assume more of this responsibility in the contact lens wearer. Also, the aqueous layer cools the eye as it evaporates.

Some eyes may be deficient in tear volume or composition, causing severe problems in contact lens wear. For example, if there is too little of the aqueous layer, the gas exchange will be too far below normal; or because of a faulty supply of mucin, the tears, though sufficient, may not spread evenly over the cornea.

A perfect illustration of this problem is the young woman referred to me because she suffered from red, itchy eyes every time she attempted to wear contact lenses. At first an allergic reaction to the lens solutions was a possibility; so was an infection. However, after probing into her medical history it was determined that the birth control pills she was taking caused a deficiency in tear production. Further examination proved indeed that her eyes were very dry. She decided that contact lens wear was important enough for her to switch to another method of birth control. Soon after the changeover, the eyes became less dry and contact lens wear became comfortable.

The eyelids, to continue the camera metaphor, could be compared to a lens cap that protects from dust and scratches. Eyelids do that and more: through the blinking mechanism, they spread tears evenly over the cornea, enabling them to do their job of cleaning, lubricating, and pumping new tears to the cornea, thus enriching the oxygen supply and removing the carbon dioxide.

Eyelashes (cilia) add further protection by acting as a barrier that prevents larger airborne particles from reaching the surface of the eye.

WHAT IS 20/20 VISION?

You've probably heard that people who see "normally" have "20/20 vision." But what exactly does that familiar label refer to? It's simply a shorthand way of indicating how sharply your eyes can focus on a certain size letter at a distance of 20 feet. The first 20 refers to the distance at which the test is being given; the second 20 refers to the distance at which you should be able to clearly see letters of that size. So if you have 20/20 vision, you can see the letters in a specified line on the eye chart at 20 feet; if you have 20/40 vision, you can see clearly at 20 feet what someone with normal vision would see at 40 feet; and if you're 20/150, you see at 20 feet what you should be able to see 150 feet away. (There are some rare cases of 20/10 vision, which is better than average; they can read movie marquees and road signs before anyone else.)

WHEN THINGS GO WRONG—REFRACTIVE ERRORS

The lens in your eye can only adjust so much in an effort to bring objects into focus. When the eye can't focus properly, there are four basic conditions that may be the cause. These are called *refractive errors* (myopia, hyperopia, astigmatism, and presbyopia). Luckily, all are correctible with contact lenses or spectacles. Most of these refractive errors are a result of heredity.

Nearsightedness (Myopia). This occurs when the eyeball is too long for the lens's focal capacity. The patient's cornea and lens focus the image of a distant object in front of the retina, so vision is blurry except when looking at nearby objects. Myopia affects one quarter of the world and seems to be on the rise, though it's a mystery why. Most contact lens wearers are myopes.

Farsightedness (Hyperopia). This occurs when the eyeball is too short. As a result the lens of the eye can't bring near objects into focus by the time the image reaches the retina. (Theoretically the focal point is behind the retina.) Therefore close objects are blurry, and distant objects are clear. In mild cases distant objects are seen clearly enough so constant visual correction is not required. In severe cases distance vision may also be affected, so the hyperope needs to wear some form of vision correction constantly; these are more likely candidates for contact lenses, though the percentage is far lower than for myopia.

Astigmatism. This is a bit harder to understand. Astigmatism is a refractive error that usually results from a cornea that isn't perfectly round, but shaped more like a football than the usual basketball shape. Imagine the cornea as a dome divided into segments by lines drawn across its surface that intersect at its center, like the segments of an orange. The normal eye, with a spherical cornea, has the same curved lines all around. The astigmatic's aspherical cornea has differently curved lines like one half of a lemon, with any given line either flatter or steeper than the one perpendicular to it. Therefore the vertical and horizontal components of both near and far images can't focus together. As a result the image appears blurry. Occasionally the crystalline lens—not the cornea—is at fault in astigmatism. Astigmatism is very common and often occurs in addition to myopia or hyperopia.

Presbyopia. This is part of the aging process (usually after the age of forty) and is due to the gradual loss of elasticity of the crystalline lens of the eye. As the lens loses its flexibility, one has more and more difficulty focusing on nearby objects. You'll know your eyes are "getting old" if your arms seem too short when you read, or if you have trouble performing close-up tasks like threading a needle. Presbyopia will occur in addition to the "Big Three"—myopia, hyperopia, and astigmatism—but

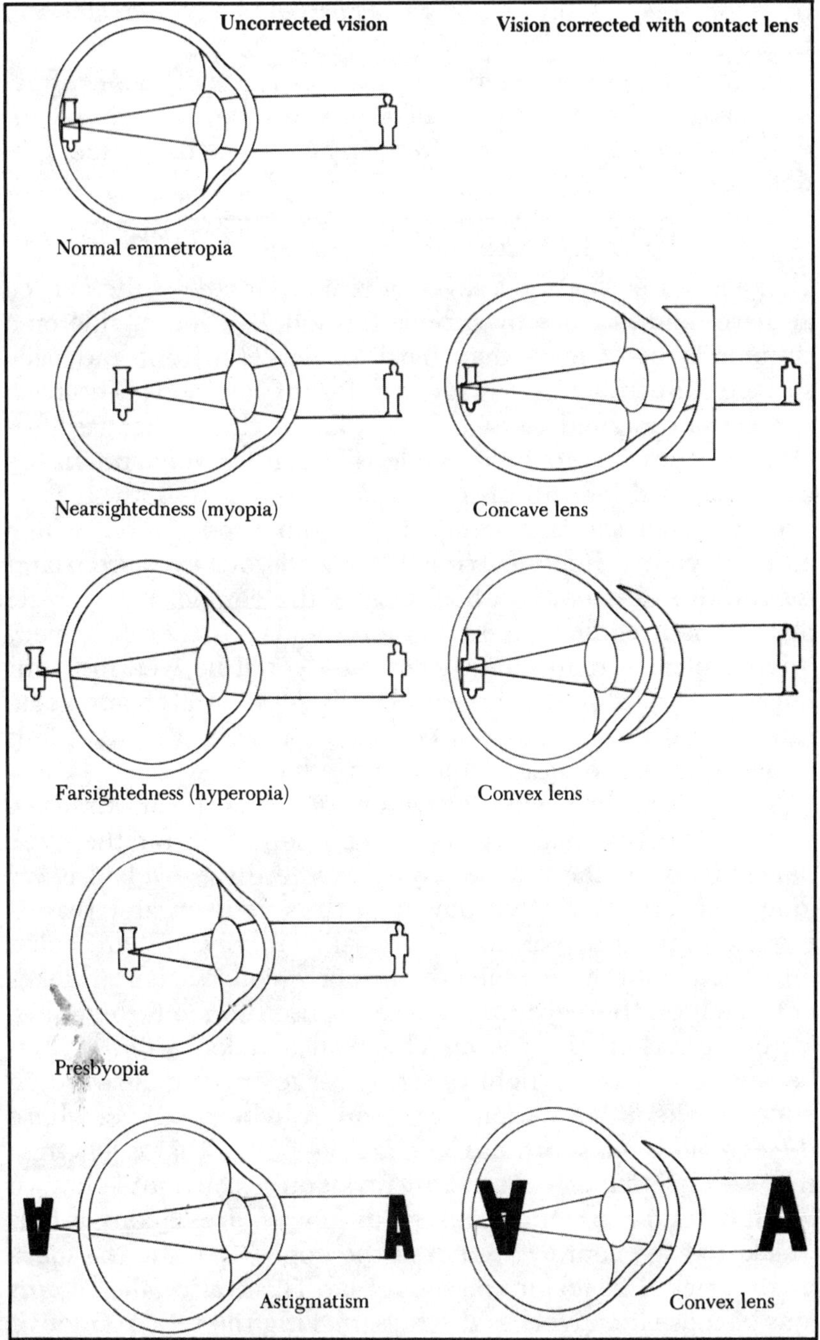

Figure 3. Refractive Errors

pure presbyopes only require a correction during close-up tasks.

Nearly half our population has one or more of these refractive errors. Fortunately all of them can be corrected with eyeglasses or contact lenses. In nearly all cases the contact lens does it better.

HOW DO CONTACT LENSES WORK?

Contact lenses float on a layer of tears that covers the cornea and are held in place by surface tension. Soft lenses ride on a thinner layer of tears than hard lenses. The front and back surfaces of contact lenses serve different functions. The back surface is designed to fit the contour of the cornea itself as closely as possible to make the lens fit comfortably and, in the case of a hard lens, to provide a new, round, smooth surface. The front surface is designed to fit your prescription, which corrects your refractive error. How well your eyes are examined and measured, and how closely the contact lenses' size, fit, and shape come to these measurements are, therefore, very important factors in how successfully you'll be wearing your lenses. Everything is done with highly sophisticated and accurate optical instruments, in combination with a contact lens practitioner's experience and knowledge.

As shown in the smaller drawings for each type of refractive error, corrective lenses work by compensating for the eye's deficiencies. In the case of myopia, where the eyeball is too long, the total refractive power of the eye is greater than is required for an eye of normal length. The rays of light come into focus before they reach the retina. A concave lens (thicker at the edges, thinner in the center) is used to focus the image farther back, on the retina. This is also called a *minus* lens because it causes the light rays to diverge or bend outward, in effect weakening the total refraction. A hyperopic eye, where the eyeball is too short, has a refractive power that is less than that of a normal eye. The light rays don't focus until they've fallen behind the retina. This condition requires a convex lens (thicker at the center, thinner at the edges) to bring the focus point forward, so it lands on the retina. This is also called a *plus* lens because it converges the rays, making the total refractive power of the eye stronger. A presbyopic eye also requires a convex lens, which is often prescribed in the form of bifocals. (Yes, they can make bifocal contact lenses.) Astigmatism requires special curves in the lenses that focus the rays of light at a specific axis.

A contact lens, with the layer of tears trapped beneath it, works by canceling out the refractive error. In effect it becomes another layer of the eye. It may be considered a prosthesis, or artificial body part, which actually becomes an integral part of the wearer's optical system. Since it is placed directly on the living eye, it must go far beyond having the correct prescription; it must fit the cornea well enough not to interfere with the normal metabolism of the eye.

Of primary concern is the amount of oxygen that reaches the cornea, which is normally supplied by the air and the tears in exchange for waste carbon dioxide. Since every lens in use acts as a barrier against both the tears and the air reaching the cornea, contact lenses are designed and fitted to overcome this problem. Though the eye can adapt somewhat, a too-diminished gas exchange radically alters the metabolism of the cornea and its health will suffer. The primary effect of such suffocation is *edema,* a swelling of the cornea that can be likened to a blister on your skin. Edema may lead to more serious injuries to the delicate cornea, and is the most prevalent of all contact lens side effects. The race to design a better contact lens is now largely a battle against the oxygen barrier.

In designing a contact lens, there are two ways to increase the gas exchange and prevent or reduce edema:

THROUGH THE TEARS

With each blink the eye trades new tears for old. By improving the tear-pump mechanism, more spent, carbon dioxide–rich tears are alternately forced out from under the lens and more fresh, oxygen-rich tears are injected.

In order for the tear pump to work, contact lenses must be able to move slightly with each blink. Both soft lenses and hard lenses float on a thin layer of tears.

THROUGH THE LENS ITSELF

In gas-permeable lenses special materials (silicone and cellulose acetate butyrate) allow gases to pass through the lens material. In soft contact lenses the lenses themselves absorb the tears in which the oxygen is dissolved and transmitted to the cornea.

Ideally, both mechanisms should operate because even in gas-permeable lenses the oxygen transmission is not 100 percent. In addition to supplying oxygen, tears also meet other requirements of the cornea, such as lubricating the corneal surface, flushing away foreign bodies, and preventing infection because of its lysozyme content.

COMPARISON OF OXYGEN PERMEABILITY

Conventional hard lenses (including modified)	5 percent or less
Conventional soft lenses	40 percent
Gas-permeable lenses	80 percent
Extended-wear lenses (soft)	75 percent
Silicone lenses	100 percent

These percentages are approximate averages; the amount varies according to various factors, such as the thickness of the lens material (which varies from prescription to prescription) and the cleanliness of the lens.

In conventional hard lenses oxygen is supplied mainly through the tear pump. In some cases *fenestrations,* or tiny holes drilled into the lenses, can make them somewhat gas permeable because air can pass through the holes. Making lenses smaller and thinner increases the tear supply; so can the use of drops of artificial tears. As frivolous as this sounds, proper blinking is crucial for proper tear flow and contact lens comfort.

HOW CONTACT LENSES ARE MADE

Contact lenses are made by companies that have the special equipment and experience needed to manufacture these precise optical devices. Because the tiniest deviation results in a lens that doesn't fit, the industry employs a highly accurate, computerized technology. There are three basic methods used to produce most contact lenses, but new techniques are being tested by researchers whose goal is to produce the lenses even more accurately—and at lower expense. Regardless of the method used, manufacture is guided, in the case of hard lenses, by the American National Standards Institute; for soft and gas-permeable lenses, the Food and Drug Administration must give its approval before they can be released to the general public.

In the *lathe-cut* method buttons of plastic are cut on precision machinery, and then the surface and edges are finished and polished smooth. Both hard and soft lenses can be made using this process, since a soft lens remains hard until it is hydrated after manufacture. For the *molded* process the company produces a molded lens by pouring the liquid plastic into a specific mold under high pressure. After molding, the lenses still need to be polished. *Spin-casting* is another method used to create soft lenses. While in liquid form, a precise amount of plastic is spun in a mold. The shape and diameter of the mold, the amount of plastic injected, the spin-speed and surface tension can be varied to form lenses of the specific corrective power needed. Though these lenses are limited in variations, the process results in a smooth surface that doesn't need to be polished and can be accurately duplicated. (Minute scratches on the surface of the lenses produced by the other two methods are occasionally a problem.)

THE CASE FOR CONTACT LENSES

In the past there was no choice but to wear spectacles to correct poor vision. These days there is a choice: Any form of poor vision that can be corrected by glasses can also be corrected by contact lenses, and usually more effectively.

WHAT'S WRONG WITH EYEGLASSES?

Admittedly, eyeglasses do have a few advantages over contacts. They're easy to get used to and easy to care for, but if you've ever worn glasses, you're all too familiar with these annoying disadvantages:

They May Not Be Flattering. Behind thick glasses, which correct large refractive errors, eyes look abnormally big or small. Glasses also tend to hide the natural beauty of the eyes, one of the most important and communicative features of the face. In spite of designer frames (which go out of style) most people look better without glasses.

They're Heavy and Uncomfortable. The pressure of the frames resting on the bridge of the nose and behind the ear can create red marks, indentations, and discomfort.

They Slip. When you look down or engage in physical activity, glasses tend to slip down your nose. If the lenses are thick and relatively heavy, and/or the frame is the type that's easily stretched out of shape, you can actually get a headache when the muscles behind the ears contract in an effort to halt the slippage.

They Get Wet, Scratched, and Smudged. Droplets of rain, perspiration, oily secretion from the fingers, and all kinds of "dirt" can collect on the lens surface, causing blurred vision. Plastic lenses are particularly prone to scratching.

They Fog Up. When you go from a cold environment to a warmer one—for example, from the outdoors on a cold day to the inside—glasses tend to steam up, obliterating your vision.

They're Bulky. Carrying glasses around all day is a nuisance and inconvenience. It means bulging pockets instead of a neat, trim appearance; or extra-large handbags or shoulder bags to provide added space for glasses and their cases. Though contact lens wearers do need to bring along a carrying case and selection of solutions, these tiny items can't compare with bulky eyeglasses, if one uses the specially designed travel-size versions.

They're Easily Lost or Forgotten. Once they're off your face, glasses are easily misplaced or simply "left behind" (consciously or subconsciously).

Their Frames Can Break. How often have you (or someone you know) sat on a pair of glasses? Or lost the little screw that connects the sidepiece with the front?

No Side Vision. Your peripheral vision isn't corrected since the size of the lens is limited. You must look through the center of the lens for the sharpest image. In addition the frame is always in the way and blocks part of your view. For clearest vision, when you want to look up, down, or to the side, you must move your whole head while keeping your eyes looking straight ahead.

The "Window Effect." With eyeglasses you always feel as though you're looking at things through a window, as if something separates you from the real world. A contributing factor may be the fact that spectacles, even though transparent, slightly reduce the amount of light reaching the eye, giving you a dimmer view of the world.

They Distort Objects. The thicker the lens, the more distortion there is in size and shape of objects, especially if you do not look through the direct center of a spectacle lens.

They Get in the Way. Try kissing, or lying on your side, or using a camera, while wearing glasses. Moreover, though it's difficult to apply makeup while wearing glasses, it's often impossible without them.

WHAT'S RIGHT WITH CONTACT LENSES?

Since contact lenses rest directly—and nearly invisibly—on a thin layer of tears over the cornea, there are many advantages:

You Look Better. This is thc greatest single reason people switch from glasses to contacts. (According to a recent survey conducted by Health Products Research, Inc., and cited in the April 1980 issue of *Contact Lens Forum,* more than 77 percent of contact lens wearers polled were primarily concerned with appearance.) There are no unflattering frames to obscure and change the appearance of your face, nor thick lenses to enlarge or diminish your eyes. Contact lenses have been called "invisible glasses" that allow the natural beauty of your eyes, eyelids, and eyelashes to be seen by everyone, and you'll be able to communicate better with them.

You See Better. There's none of the distortion of objects that can occur when you wear thick eyeglasses. In most cases refractive errors are corrected better with contacts, and some myopes see better than 20/20: 20/15 or even 20/10. About 66 percent of the contact lens wearers in the above survey said improved vision correction helped them make the switch from spectacles.

You Feel Better. Looking better and seeing better bring an undeniable psychological lift. Many contact lens wearers say they feel less inhibited and more confident; that they don't hide behind their glasses anymore; that they perform better socially and professionally because contacts give them "a new lease on life." In fact contacts allow about 4 percent more light to be transmitted than glasses do, so the world not only seems brighter—it is! I've seen dozens of shy, seemingly inhibited spectacle-wearing patients who, after adapting to a pair of contact lenses, miraculously changed into outgoing, self-confident people. This transformation can honestly be compared to a drug-free "high."

They Don't Fog Up. Contacts don't get steamed up when you come in from the cold. And moisture, in the form of perspiration or rain, is actually beneficial to contact lenses and helps keep the vision clear, so there's no slipping down a sweaty or greasy nose, and you won't dread being caught in the rain.

They're Convenient. You'll avoid the nuisance and bulkiness that goes with carrying and wearing glasses. The contact lens carrying case you may need to take with you is tiny compared to a case for a pair of glasses.

No More Headaches. Because they don't slip around, properly fitted contact lenses are comfortable and don't cause the headaches precipitated by tense scalp muscles, or pinching behind the ears.

Good Side Vision. Because the field of vision isn't limited by frames and contact lenses move with your eyes, contact lenses provide full peripheral vision. This is especially useful in sports, driving, and other jobs and leisure activities requiring good side vision.

They're Great for Active People. No matter how rugged the sport, contacts are safe and give you more freedom than glasses. (Under certain conditions you can even swim while wearing them.) Your new, improved peripheral vision gives the game a whole new dimension. And if you see better, you'll play better and win more often.

They Do More than Correct Refractive Errors. Tinted lenses can subtly enhance the natural color of your eyes. And special cosmetic lenses do wonders for those people, including actors and actresses, who have small, bland-colored eyes. These unique lenses are opaque in the area that covers the iris and can be colored to suit your specifications. (The central area is transparent to maintain vision.) Now anyone can have gorgeous, vibrant eyes colored blue, green, or even violet to rival Elizabeth Taylor's famous orbs. On a more serious note, special lenses called X Chrom lenses help people who are color-blind, and prosthetic lenses can disguise disfigured eyes.

You Can See Clearly from the Minute You Wake up till the Minute You Go to Sleep. With the new extended-wear lenses, you can even sleep while wearing them. As one happy wearer says, "It's almost like having an eye transplant!"

ARE YOU A GOOD CONTACT LENS CANDIDATE?

By now you're probably sold on the idea of contacts. They seem to be the answer to all your prayers. Before you throw away your glasses and plunk down your hard-earned cash, remember: To get any contact lens is easy. To get the right contact lens for your eyes requires motivation, choosing a qualified eye practitioner, and having the commitment to follow the instructions for the care and handling of your valuable investment. Wearing contact lenses is in some ways like owning and driving a car. Though it undoubtedly makes life easier and more pleasant, you also will need to find a parking space, get the car inspected and registered, and be able to maintain it and handle it reasonably well in order to get the most out of it. Not everyone is a skilled or responsible driver, or is willing to spend the time and money a car requires. It's estimated that 99 percent of those who want contacts can wear them if fitted by an expert. But lenses aren't for everyone. How do you know you're not in that 1 percent who doesn't qualify? Just keep the following points in mind.

No Motivation. If you don't have a real desire to wear contact lenses, you won't be able to do so no matter how comfortable they are or how well you see with them. If your mother or boyfriend or spouse desperately wants you to try contacts—and you couldn't care less—listen to yourself. The best candidates by far are those who need to wear their glasses constantly for good vision, and have strong motivation. On the other hand those who have reasonably good vision without glasses, or who don't particularly care about wearing lenses, make poor candidates.

Fear. Almost everyone is squeamish to some degree about putting anything in their eyes. Over 26 percent of those who don't want to switch from glasses to contacts cite this reason in the study by Health Products Research, Inc. But most people can overcome this obstacle with the proper training and practice—if they are sufficiently motivated.

Poor Fit. I can't stress this too much. Exact fitting by an expert contact lens practitioner is crucial to your comfort, to the health of your eye, and to good vision . . . and therefore to successful contact lens wear. No matter how motivated or fearless you are, if the lens doesn't fit, you won't be able to wear it. Discomfort and poor vision usually send the wearer back to the fitter. But subtle symptoms of poor fit may be accepted as a fact of life by the unaware contact lens patient. Lenses that slip around or pop out with unusual frequency are examples. I recall one woman whose contact lenses often popped out when she laughed. She had erroneously assumed that the problem was uncorrectable and due to her peculiar prescription, rather than to poor fit. She felt foolish bringing it up to her eye doctor, but when she did, she was refitted. Now she can laugh herself silly, but the lenses stay in place.

Bad Hygiene. If you are careless about cleanliness and won't follow the specific hygienic rules about the care and handling of lenses, you shouldn't wear them. Lenses worn under dirty conditions can lead to eye irritation and infection.

Occupation. Some vocations create hazardous conditions for contact lens wearers because the work area has air polluted by chemical vapors and sprays. Beauticians and chemists are two professions that fall into this category; they can, of course, wear their lenses when away from work. Anyone exposed to chemical fumes, vapors, intense heat, molten metals, or atmospheres with high dust levels should not wear contact lenses.

Physical Handicaps. If you have severe arthritis, tremors, or a similar condition, you may have difficulties handling contact lenses. They are small, relatively delicate articles, and they require a certain amount of manual dexterity to handle without mishaps. (Of course extended-wear contacts could be the answer to this problem.)

Psychological Factors. There are some people who are emotionally or mentally unfit to cope with contact lenses; these include nervous, fidgety types, those who are unstable and unable to follow a routine, and those with low IQs.

Age. Extreme youth or very old age can sometimes preclude contact lens wear because of a lack of motor skills, which may not yet have developed or may have degenerated. Motivation may also be lacking in these members of the population, as well as a willingness to comply with the strict hygienic routine. However, new contact lenses and a doctor with expertise in the contact lens field can overcome these problems. In fact, children as young as seven years of age make excellent candidates because they tend to follow directions well and look to the eye doctor as a teacher figure. However, they must be motivated, have a sense of proper hygiene, and have good motor control.

Allergies. If you suffer from hay fever, you may notice increased eye irritation during the "peak season." You may have to stop wearing your lenses during that time, or go on a reduced schedule. On the other hand some lens wearers point out that they feel less irritation because contacts are a deterrent to rubbing the eyes to relieve the itching, which can in fact worsen the condition. Occasionally I run across a patient who is allergic to the solutions used in conjunction with the lenses; but this is usually solved simply by switching brands or employing different cleaning methods.

Eye Disorders. Any active infection of the eye and the surrounding tissues is a contraindication to wearing contact lenses. If you suffer from chronic or recurring eye infections, contact lenses are not for you. Of course, a fleeting eye infection simply means you should forego contact lens wear until that condition clears up. A few people have unusually "dry eyes"—meaning the eye doesn't produce tears in sufficient quantity to make contact lenses comfortable. This condition usually remains unknown until the ophthalmologist tests you for it. A slightly dry eye may pose some problems, especially for soft lens wearers, but special lubricating eye drops or medication may solve this problem.

THE WHO AND WHERE OF BUYING CONTACT LENSES

There are three types of eye professionals who, by law, are qualified to fit contact lenses: ophthalmologists, optometrists, and opticians. Unfortunately, most people aren't sure of the differences among them.

OPHTHALMOLOGIST (M.D.)

This is a medical doctor who specializes in the diagnosis, treatment, and surgery of the eye. He or she prescribes whatever eye treatment you may need, including prescriptions for glasses and the fitting of contact lenses. All ophthalmologists can provide a prescription for glasses and contact lenses; half of them also specialize in *fitting* contact lenses. Ophthalmologists spend a minimum of eight years training after college: After four years of general medical study at an approved medical school, they then spend an additional one to two years in general internship, and at least three more years in special ophthalmologic residency training at an approved hospital.

OPTOMETRIST (D.O.)

A doctor of optometry spends four years in specialized optometric study after college. He or she is trained to examine the eyes, to prescribe, and to fit glasses and contact lenses. There are about twice as many optometrists as there are ophthalmologists, and a large proportion of them fit and dispense contact lenses.

OPTICIAN

An eye practitioner who is trained (usually for two years in an optician's school) and is authorized to fill the prescriptions of ophthalmologists and optometrists (but not prescribe himself). In some states he or she may fit contact lenses.

If you have decided that you would like to wear contact lenses, I strongly recommend that you first go to an ophthalmologist for a medical eye examination. The next step is to choose the contact lens specialist (it may be the same ophthalmologist) who will fit and order your contact lenses, as well as provide you with follow-up care. For this it's best to go to an ophthalmologist or optometrist in private practice who specializes in contact lenses. He or she is probably the most trustworthy, reliable, and knowledgeable source, and though you may spend more initially than if you went to a different type of eye specialist, this is one case where *you get what you pay for.* An ophthalmologist can best detect any present, past, or latent eye diseases and potential problems of the eye that might not only interfere with contact lens wear, but may affect your vision in general. By examining your eyes he can also detect signs and symptoms of diseases elsewhere in the body. Diseases that exhibit early ocular symptoms include diabetes, high blood pressure, arteriosclerosis, kidney disease, blood disease, and certain neurologic disorders. Thus you not only save money by not buying lenses that you won't be able to wear successfully, but you might also be saving your sight—and perhaps even your life. Even if your ophthalmologist doesn't fit contact lenses himself, you should go to him for your initial medical ocular examination. He will then refer you to an eye practitioner who is specially trained to fit contact lenses. In all cases you should remain under the ophthalmologist's care, supervision, and responsibility. An optometrist, although lacking the training of a four-year medical school, does have the background training to diagnose many eye disorders. However, he cannot treat any ocular diseases.

Then there's the matter of prescription and fit. You simply stand a better chance for a successful fit under the care of a private contact lens specialist, be he an ophthalmologist or optometrist, because of his virtually unlimited choice of lenses. The contact lens specialist isn't committed to any one manufacturer, and can therefore choose exactly the lens which will best suit your individual needs. Having access to hundreds of lenses manufactured by many different companies is important because no one brand can fit everyone; all brands were *not* created equal.

There are some "optical stores," on the other hand, which may buy large quantities of contact lenses from one or two manufacturers in order to obtain volume discounts that they can pass on to their customers at low markup. While you may benefit from lower prices because of the large inventory, it may be the store's policy to try to fit you with one of their stock lenses because of their financial commitment. You forfeit having the choice of all the types of lenses in order to choose the one that specifically meets your own visual correction needs. It is unlikely that these stores hire ophthalmologists. Therefore the all-important initial medical exam is missing. Usually cursory eye exams are often the rule as well as a quick and sometimes inadequate instruction session. These shortcuts are two of the most often-cited reasons for contact lens dropouts. In one survey (completed in 1979 and reported in *Contact Lens Forum* by Dr. Robert J. Morrison, a Harrisburg, Pennsylvania, ophthalmologist), 92 percent of past contact lens failures were refitted successfully when they went to optometrists and ophthalmologists who specialized in contact lenses. In another survey of contact lens dropouts (also conducted in 1978–1979 and reported in the same article) 78 percent of the patients had gone to low-cost dispensers and almost that many admitted they hadn't been thoroughly briefed on the importance of the meticulous care and handling the lenses required. Should you balk at the higher cost, remember that quality *seems* expensive at first. But when you can wear a comfortable pair of lenses that provides excellent vision, it is cheaper in the long run. What is the difference between a bargain contact lens and an expensive pair? You can liken the plastic of a contact lens to a bolt of fine silk. In the hands of a mass-production firm, the silk can be fashioned into an inexpensive shirt. By contrast, in the hands of a fine couturier, the raw silk material becomes an exquisitely made, well-fitting, good-looking article of clothing that, although expensive, you will wear with pride for many years. The silk, though it may be of high quality to begin with, accounts for only a fraction of the cost of the final product. The inexpensive shirt that may fit poorly and not look so great may turn out to be no bargain if not worn. On the other hand that expensive silk shirt that you wear frequently will, in reality, be the bargain!

I have personally examined many patients who bought "bargain lenses." A great number of these were wearing poorly fitting contact lenses that caused poor vision and in some cases eye irritation. Not only did they have to discard those lenses and suffer a loss of money, but some had potentially serious eye problems related to those lenses. In the words of one (now) satisfied wearer: "I only paid eighty-nine dollars for my soft lenses, but I had to go back *five times* with additional cost for refitting before they managed to find a comfortable lens for my right eye. In between visits I was in agony because the lens in that eye didn't fit right. During each visit I felt as though they really didn't want to bother with me, and I had the sneaking suspicion that the eye exam wasn't all it should have been." Even if you should by chance obtain a pair that fits the shape of your cornea, the prescription may be off, as this bargain hunter discovered: "I went to one of those ninety-nine-dollar-special storefronts. The contacts seemed comfortable enough, but I ended up wearing my glasses most of the time anyway because I could see better with them . . . a year of sporadic contact lens wear later, I realized this was silly. After a proper examination the eye doctor discovered the contacts had the wrong prescription all along!" Nor should the contact lens wearer take a doctor's prescription to a storefront operation and expect to get completely satisfactory lenses. The importance of correctly fitted contacts cannot be exaggerated. The eye doctor, or the eye practitioner he recommends, is the person best qualified to supply you with the correct contact lenses.

Of course, there are some patients who have a high tolerance for pain and can accept almost any type of lens, or who don't mind less-than-perfect vision. Nevertheless, intelligent consumers will demand excellent vision and comfort from their contact lenses. The perfect contact lens requires time, patience, and expertise that you can only find in the hands of an expert professional eye practitioner.

The difference between a pair of cheap lenses and an expensive pair lies not so much in the lenses themselves—it lies in the professional behind the lenses. You "buy" years of experience and professional service along with those little plastic discs. To repeat, an expert practitioner doesn't attempt to make the eye fit the lens; he *fits the lens to the eye!* The eye always comes first. This important philosophy among contact lens practitioners can spell the difference between a successful and an unsuccessful contact lens wearer. Not all practitioners, however, are perfect. If you've been told "you can't wear contact lenses" or if you're not completely happy with the pair you have, consider going elsewhere for a second opinion. Patients have adopted this practice for many other medical matters, and buying a pair of contact lenses should not be any different.

When you consult a private ophthalmologist or optometrist who specializes in contact lenses, you'll be fitted more accurately and with greater ease. Instead of having a pair (or two!) of ill-fitting, inaccurately prescribed lenses lying dormant in the dresser drawer, you'll be wearing comfortable lenses that provide excellent vision. Follow-up care will be of high quality as well. Correcting problems of poor fit, discomfort, and faulty vision; maintaining the health of the eyes; replacing damaged or lost lenses; switching to new improved lenses, and so on are the hallmarks of care that only an expert contact lens practitioner can provide. He will never forget the criteria for successful contact lens fitting: long-term, full-time comfortable wear, with good vision and *healthy eyes.* Remember, you only have one pair of eyes. So please don't take them for granted. They're responsible for an estimated 80 percent of the information that your five senses tell you about the world you live in. A durable but sensitive organ, your eyes are irreplaceable. Badly fitted lenses may cause permanent damage, so economize elsewhere.

WHERE TO FIND A GOOD CONTACT LENS SPECIALIST

OPHTHALMOLOGIST

• Through word-of-mouth of friends, relatives, and neighbors who are satisfied contact lens wearers. This is no guarantee that you'll be as pleased as they are, but the chances are good.

• Through recommendation from your family physician.

• From your local medical society, which has a list of well-regarded ophthalmologists specializing in contact lenses.

• From the eye department of a hospital or medical center.

• From the *Contact Lens Association of Ophthalmologists,* 2620 Jean Street, New Orleans, Louisiana 70115.

OPTOMETRISTS

• Through word-of-mouth.

• From the *American Optometric Association,* Communications Division, 243 North Lindberg Boulevard, St. Louis, Missouri 63141.

• Through colleges of optometry.

OPTICIANS

• Through word-of-mouth.

• Through schools of opticianary.

• From the *Opticians Association of America,* 1250 Connecticut Avenue, N.W., Washington, D.C. 20036.

• From the *Contact Lens Society of America,* First National Bank Building, 167 West Main Street, Lexington, Kentucky 40507.

CHAPTER TWO

LIVING WITH CONTACT LENSES

WHAT'S IN STORE?

Once you've found a contact lens physician and have decided to go ahead and determine whether you're a likely candidate for contact lenses, you should know a bit about what's in store for you. Often a person may be sold on the idea without realizing what's involved, namely: You'll need a thorough medical eye examination and contact lens fitting. Then you'll have to go through a period of adaptation, and adhere to a wearing schedule. You may undergo frequent follow-up visits; you'll need to become proficient at, and devote a certain amount of time to, the care and handling of the lenses. You will have initial costs as well as maintenance costs.

THE MEDICAL EYE EXAMINATION

Vision is a dynamic, changing process that is highly individualized. No one sees exactly the same as you do. No two eyes—even your right eye compared with your left—are quite the same. Nor do they remain the same as you go through life.

Though the eye is quite durable, it's also an irreplaceable, delicate, sensitive, and highly sophisticated organ. Your eye is directly connected to your brain by the optic nerve and is closely related to other systems of your body. It shouldn't be considered independently, and before you walk off with a pair of contact lenses you should undergo a complete *medical* eye examination by an ophthalmologist.

Such an exam is much more than a simple mechanical test of your eye as an optical instrument. It determines what prescription you'll need. It also determines whether you'll be able to wear contact lenses safely and comfortably, and reveals clues that form a picture of your optical health and your physical condition in general. It also yields the measurements needed to "fit" you with the right pair of lenses—these measurements must be extremely accurate if you're going to be comfortable wearing lenses. To do all this, your eye doctor uses a variety of instruments and techniques that may seem baffling and mysterious to the potential contact lens consumer. Space-age technology has invaded ophthalmology, and your eye physician's examining rooms may resemble the inside of a spaceship; the instruments approximate cousins of *Star Wars* character R2D2, with futuristic beeps and digital readouts. Whether your doctor has the latest in equipment or not, the examination can be a fascinating process if you let it; and you should feel free to pepper him with questions.

History. This first step may seem casual and unscientific, but it's very important. Your eye doctor will ask you "Why are you here?" and discuss with you your motivation, occupation, leisure activities, systemic diseases and medications, eye diseases and medications, and allergies, complaints about your vision, whether you get headaches, and whether you've worn contacts before, what type they were and any problems you had while wearing them. (If you do wear contact lenses, you should keep them out of your eyes at least twenty-four hours before your exam, though seventy-two hours is preferable.)

Refraction. This step determines the prescription your lenses will need to correct whatever refractive error—nearsightedness, farsightedness, astigmatism, or presbyopia—you may have. We've come a long way from the days when a simple wall eye chart sufficed. Nowadays the doctor usually first instills special eye drops that dilate your pupils before using the two instruments, the *Phoroptor* and the *retinoscope,* to come up with your lens prescription.

First comes the Phoroptor, that familiar contraption that makes the examinee look like the ultimate bug-eyed Martian. As you gaze at the eye chart (projected on the wall), the physician tries out several lens combinations, repeatedly asking you "which is better, first or second?" Out of its billions of possible

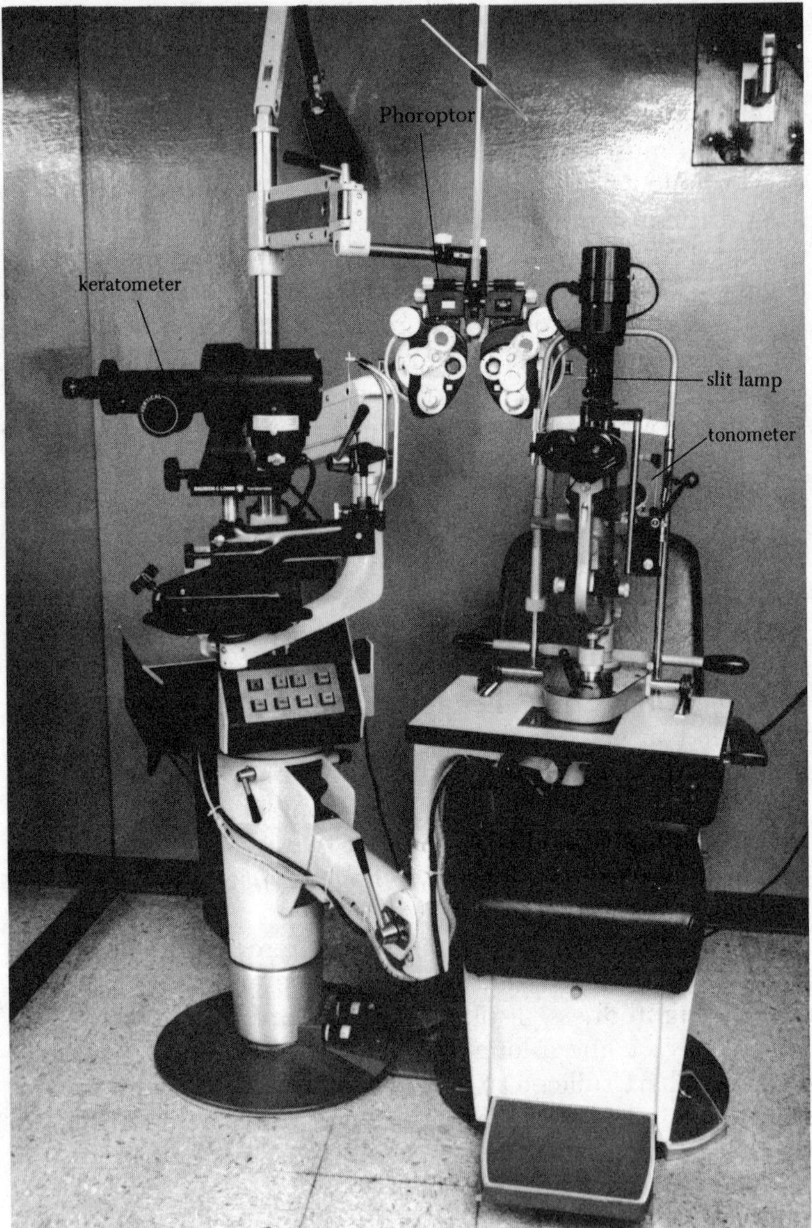

Figure 4. Before being fitted for a pair of contact lenses, you should have a complete medical eye examination by an ophthalmologist. Shown in this office are many of the instruments explained in the text, including a Phoroptor, a keratometer, a slit lamp, and a tonometer. *Photo: George Janoff*

lens combinations, the examiner determines and fine-tunes your prescription. After this subjective test (*you're* judging which lens corrects the best), the results are read off the Phoroptor in order to check the prescription by doing an objective test for refraction. As your eyes gaze at a distant target through the prescription in the Phoroptor, the doctor peers into your eyes with the retinoscope. Through the dilated pupils the light of the retinoscope creates a measurable shadow and light movement on your retina, which enables him to check the accuracy of the prescription.

Curvature of the Cornea. Using a *keratometer,* an optical scanning device, the ophthalmologist determines the exact "topography" of the cornea. A system of mirrors measures the horizontal and vertical meridians of the cornea. This determines the steepness or flatness of the cornea and its degree of corneal astigmatism, an important part of the overall refractive error picture, and instrumental in determining whether you need a hard or soft lens.

Muscle Range and Coordination. How well do your eyes work together? Do they point to and focus at various distances equally? How well do you judge distance and space (depth perception, or stereopsis)? To find out, the eye doctor uses a muscle light and special prisms.

Outer and Middle Layers of the Eye. Next comes the *slit lamp,* an electrical microscope that lights up and magnifies your eyelids, cornea, iris, lens, and fluid of your eye in order to reveal any disease, damage, inflammation, or other abnormality. A special stain called *fluorescein* is used in conjunction with a cobalt-blue filter to detect any corneal defects or abrasions not visible with the naked eye.

Inner Layers of the Eye. Through the dilated pupil, the retina and its blood vessels can be seen with an *ophthalmoscope,* which illuminates and enlarges the doctor's view. This is the point at which early signs of diabetes, hardening of the arteries, hypertension, and other general disorders of the body can be detected.

Eye Pressure. This is the "glaucoma test." The doctor anesthetizes your cornea with special eye drops, and measures the pressure of the eye fluid with a *tonometer.* Though the instrument actually touches your cornea, you don't feel a thing because of the anesthetizing eye drops. This test is especially important for anyone over the age of thirty, although it is unusual for glaucoma to occur before the age of forty. There is also a "noncontact" tonometer which utilizes a puff of air to measure the eye pressure. Although not as accurate as a tonometer, this instrument is an excellent screening device and eye drops are not instilled.

Tear Function. Tears lubricate and cleanse your eyes and also provide the cornea with oxygen. A sufficient supply of tears is a must for comfortable contact lens wear. "Dry eyes" can be countered with special eye drops if the problem is slight. To make sure it isn't a contraindication, the ophthalmologist performs the *Shirmer test:* special strips of paper placed under the lids to gauge the amount of tear production. After about five minutes the test strips are removed and the amount of tear absorption is measured and evaluated.

Visual Field. In certain instances (suspicion of glaucoma, retinal abnormalities, optic nerve disorders, neurologic disorders, headaches, and so on) a test of your peripheral vision is important. To measure your peripheral (side) vision, a special computerized instrument is used. (If you like video games, you'll love this part of the test. If you don't, the challenge may leave you a bit limp.) First each eye is tested separately, then together. Your head is kept immobile as you face a large dome, perforated with a scattering of pin-sized holes. As you gaze ahead steadily at a red-lit cross in the center of the dome, minuscule flashes of light go off through the holes, one at a time, at various distances from the center cross. Every time you see a "star" light up in this mini-planetarium, you hit a button; meanwhile the computer keeps score by adding up the correct "strikes."

Your ophthalmologist will evaluate all the information thus gleaned from all parts of the ocular examination and decide whether or not you—and your eyes—are a good candidate for contact lenses, and if so, what type. Those who "pass" the exam then go on to the next step, the contact lens fitting.

HARD OR SOFT?

Before the actual fitting, you and your ophthalmologist will sit down and discuss the type of lenses best suited to your needs and eyes. Only fifteen years ago there was only one choice: hard lenses. Today there are many types and brands of lenses available. The standard hard lenses have vastly improved, but the greatest development has been the new flexible soft lenses, which enabled many more people to wear contact lenses. But technological advancement hasn't stopped there. Now there are further refinements in the two basic types—lenses that fall somewhere in between the standard hard and soft lenses—the semisoft gas-permeable lenses that let your eyes "breathe" and are more comfortable, soft lenses that correct astigmatism, and the fabulous new super-soft, super-thin extended-wear lenses that everyone's talking about. Each has its own advantages and disadvantages, which are discussed in more detail in later chapters. For now here's a quick summary of how the two basic types compare.

Each advantage and disadvantage of the various types of contact lenses must be weighed and evaluated according to each individual case. There are still more rigid-lens wearers than soft-lens wearers, possibly because hard lenses have simply been around longer, and because lower cost, easier upkeep, and better vision override soft lenses' main advantage: comfort. On the other hand newcomers to the contact lens scene more often seem to prefer the comfort and ease of adaptation found in soft lenses. There's a contact lens created to suit just about every need. Your eye doctor is best qualified to determine which lenses will best correct your visual deficiencies and still provide comfort and safety.

Remember that the ability to wear a certain type of lens (or any contact lens at all) depends to a large degree upon the chemical makeup, amount, and behavior of the tears. Tears lubricate, cleanse, and supply the eye with nutrients. If you have too much mucus, or protein, or lipids, these deposits can cling tenaciously to the lens surface and are especially hard to remove from soft lenses. A deficiency in any component can

HARD AND SOFT LENSES COMPARED (cont.)

HARD	SOFT
Uncomfortable at first; may need 1 to 2 months to adapt to all-day wear (average 8 hours).	Comfortable almost immediately; adaptation to all-day wear is only about 1 week.
Easy care; inexpensive to keep clean; disinfection unnecessary.	Cleaning more involved and slightly more expensive; disinfection necessary.
Durable, long life—some up to 10 years.	More delicate, less durable—most need replacement after 2 years.
Excellent visual acuity; consistently clear, sharp image for all refractive errors.	Less satisfactory correction, especially in astigmatism.
Lenses must be removed and cleaned when dirt or dust gets between them and cornea.	Dust and dirt rarely get under lenses.
Vision may be temporarily blurry after removal ("spectacle blur").	No spectacle blur.
Once adapted, should be worn same number of hours each day.	Can wear intermittently for special reasons (evening, sports, etc.).
Eyelid sensation with each blink.	No eyelid discomfort.
Tend to pop out or move off center.	Less chance of popping out or moving around eye—best for sports.

render the eyes too "dry" for successful contact lens wear, even if the watery layer is sufficient. That's why you may be able to wear soft lenses without a hitch, but your best friend can't. Then, too, some eyes need a greater amount of oxygen than others and some eyes fail to adapt to the lower metabolism imposed upon the eye by any contact lens. These complications often only become evident after the lenses have been worn for some time, and may take patience and a good deal of skill and expertise on the part of the eye practitioner to overcome.

THE CONTACT LENS FITTING

This is the most exciting stage for any new contact lens wearer. At last the moment has arrived when you get to know how

HARD AND SOFT LENSES COMPARED (cont.)

HARD	SOFT
Relatively low in cost.	Higher cost.
Prescription of lens can be reground to accommodate slight visual changes.	Vision change requires new lens.
Danger of overwearing and corneal damage.	Less danger of injury from overwearing.
Some side glare and reflections from edge of lens; increased sensitivity to light.	Little side glare—better for night driving; little or no increased light sensitivity.
Average daily wearing time: 8 hours.	Average daily wearing time: 14 hours.
Unaffected by atmospheric conditions; doesn't absorb foreign substances.	Can be uncomfortable in dry air; can absorb and accumulate substances such as hair spray, chemical fumes, even eye secretions.
Routinely tinted. May put dot on right lens.	Tinting is possible, but not yet routine nor widely available.
Difficult to wear with dry eyes.	Almost impossible to wear with dry eyes.
Scratches on lenses may be polished.	Scratched lens has to be discarded.

they really feel, and what a thrill it is to see—and see yourself—without glasses. If you're being refitted, you'll be anticipating increased comfort and improved vision over your old pair of lenses.

You may be surprised to learn that fitting is an art in addition to being a precise science. Contact lenses do not fit your cornea like a second skin or the way a lid fits tightly on a jar. That would prove as uncomfortable as an overly snug garment or a tight pair of shoes; it would also prove unhealthy for the cornea. Rather, the lens must float on just the right amount of tears, which must flow freely under the edge of the lens. As you've seen, the tears not only cushion the cornea like a pair of socks cushion your feet, they also clean it and provide it with vital oxygen and nutrients. You may remember the grade-school experiment whereby a glass tumbler is placed over a lit candle, forming an air-tight seal. Eventually the oxygen is consumed and the flame flickers and dies. A cornea deprived of oxygen suffers too—by becoming swollen and clouded. So a lens must fit "loosely" enough to move slightly with each blink, which allows the free exchange of oxygen and carbon dioxide in the tears to occur.

On the other hand a lens must fit snugly enough so that it doesn't slip around too much. Such slippage would result in blurred vision, possibly irritation, and a lens that may pop out. Your feet are just as unhappy in too-loose, blister-causing shoes as they are in too-tight toe-pinchers. This is where the "art" begins to come in: the fitter must seek a delicate balance between tightness and looseness to achieve optimum wear.

To facilitate the fitting the doctor will place a pair of *trial contact lenses* on your eyes. These will closely approximate your final prescription, but they are not your final contact lenses, so don't be unduly upset if your vision isn't crystal clear at this point. Since this is probably the first time you've voluntarily allowed anything solid to be placed in your eye, it may be a tense encounter. Novices should just try to relax and let the doctor do his job; soon you'll be inserting them yourself without giving it a second thought.

Fitting doesn't stop with the insertion of trial lenses. Even after measurements have been made and the most suitable lenses tried, other fitting factors come into play. A high minus lens, for instance (for myopia), tends to ride high on the eye because of the shape of the lens that the prescription dictates. A high plus lens on the other hand (for hyperopia) tends to fall slightly downward once placed on the eye. Such decentered lenses may cause discomfort in addition to less-than-perfect vision. To correct this phenomenon a lens may need to be smaller or larger, heavier or lighter, steeper or flatter, or some combination of these factors.

After about a half hour of wearing your trial lenses, the doctor will examine your eyes while the lenses are in place. In addition to testing the refraction, he will examine your eyes with the slit lamp in order to check the size and fit of the lenses in relation to the cornea.

From the information gathered from the trial lenses the

practitioner will then order the exact lenses you'll need. If you are being fitted for hard or gas-permeable contact lenses, your lenses will be "custom-made": that is, the exact prescription can be permanently carved into the plastic, as well as the exact size and curvature made for each lens. Unfortunately the time has not yet come when soft lenses are completely custom-designed for the individual, though minor modifications can be made in stock lenses that approach custom-made in fit and performance.

When your lenses have arrived, you will return to pick them up, and have them inserted and evaluated while they're in the eyes. You'll also be taught the correct way to handle, insert, and remove the lenses. Usually a highly trained technician performs this function, shows you films, and supplies you with pamphlets that instruct you in the proper procedures. Make sure that before you leave the office, you understand and have practiced these procedures. You'll also receive a wearing schedule and whatever equipment and products are required to clean and maintain your lenses. Once the technician is satisfied that you have practiced care techniques enough to have mastered them, and that you are familiar with the products, you'll be allowed to depart with your lenses.

FOLLOW-UP VISITS

After you've worn the lenses for a specified number of days, following the wearing schedule you were given, you'll report back to the doctor for the important reevaluation. He'll reexamine your eyes to test for visual acuity and fit of the lenses, as well as to ask you to discuss any questions or problems you may have. Whatever adjustments are necessary will be made then, and at any future time, until the lenses are perfect. Thereafter, six-month checkups are scheduled in order to maintain that perfection. (Of course, if any problems should arise between checkups, you should call the doctor's office immediately.)

ADAPTATION AND WEARING SCHEDULES

Once your lenses are ready for you to take home and you and your doctor are confident that you understand the principles of lens wear and care, and are proficient in their insertion, centering, and removal, you'll be given a written *wearing schedule* to follow. You might balk at the rigidity of such a schedule—so many hours the first day, so many the next, gradually increasing the wearing time over a week or two—but wearing schedules are carefully designed to help your eyes adjust to the presence of a new, plastic foreign object.

The thinner and softer the lens, and the better it fits, the more comfortable it will be. But even the thinnest hard lens and the supplest soft one will require that your eyes adapt gradually to their wear. This buildup phase has the reputation of being the least pleasant aspect of the contact lens initiation. Leery of that prospect, many a potential wearer and all too many a candidate have shied away from successful full-time wear. But the quality, quantity, and fitting techniques of contact lenses have vastly improved over the years and are still steadily improving. If you have personally tried to convert to contacts in the past and gave up, or if you have succumbed to the secondhand tales of disappointment of others, take heart. Adaptation, particularly in the case of hard lenses, still entails a certain amount of temporary discomfort. But unless you have been misfitted, it should not resemble the teary, red-eyed interludes of yore.

What is adaptation? And why do most people adapt more easily to soft lenses than to hard ones? To begin with, your eye must adjust to the simple fact that a contact lens is a foreign object. However, you shouldn't think of a contact lens the same way you think of objects such as specks of dust or eyelashes that can get into the eye and cause pain. Contact lenses are objects that float on a cushioning layer of tears and slide unnoticeably over your cornea every time you blink. They've been especially made to fit your cornea as perfectly as possible, and so minimize the foreign-body sensation. Soft lenses conform to the shape of the cornea, so the feeling of the lid bumping into the lens edge is even less.

Exactly how your eye eventually learns to live with the constant presence of a contact lens is still a mystery. Babies don't enjoy shoes or clothes when they're first put on, but eventually they adjust; well-fitted clothing feels as if it isn't there. Somehow the nerve impulses adjust and quiet down. Most of the foreign-body sensation is in the cornea (in fact it's the most sensitive part of the body). Contrary to some old wives' tales that you may have heard, the lids are not the main area of adaptation, and they do not become "callused." Think of the way a new pair of shoes might feel uncomfortable and tight at first. Later on you are not even aware that you're wearing them.

During adaptation your eyes also become used to a mild reduction in oxygen and a slight elevation in temperature. The cornea adapts by learning how to fulfill its metabolic requirements more efficiently. In conjunction with this corneal "belt-tightening" the amount of gas exchanged from the tears increases; blood vessels in the *limbus* (the border between the cornea and the sclera) pitch in by dilating so the blood flow surrounding the cornea increases. If the cornea cannot adapt sufficiently, an oxygen debt builds up, resulting in edema. The early symptoms of edema are slight and subtle. In mild cases the eyes become reddened (from dilated blood vessels), vision becomes clouded, and the lenses feel irritating. As the condition worsens, the corneal nerves gradually become less sensitive so no actual pain is felt while the lens is being worn. However, a few hours after the lens is removed, severe ocular pain occurs and may last for several hours. It's similar to what happens when your foot falls asleep in a certain position; as long as it's asleep and numb, you feel nothing. When you change position and circulation begins to be restored, the uncomfortable tingling sensation begins. Edema is the most common recurrent symptom in any contact lens specialist's practice. Several times each year I can count on an emergency call in the middle of the night from a new contact lens wearer with severe ocular pain. The history is always the same: the patient—either consciously or unconsciously—had exceeded the prescribed maximum wearing time. Typically, the pain wasn't bad at first, when the lenses were removed. But at 3:00 A.M. it was terrible. Examination always reveals corneal edema; patching and bed rest usually are enough to cure the problem.

The initial and eventual tolerance, rate, and degree of adaptation vary tremendously from patient to patient. You may belong to that fortunate group who can wear their lenses in comfort for hours from the very start; more likely you'll have to "break in" your lenses more gradually. (Similarly, few runners can—or should—complete ten miles on the first day of a training program. The mind may be willing, the muscles and lungs may even be capable, but the heart and bone structure may not be up to it.) The adaptation period takes a week or more, depending upon you and your lens type. Once adapted, most people can wear their lenses comfortably during all their waking hours.

TIPS

- During the first few days wear your lenses at home, in a quiet, tension-free environment.

- Even if the lenses feel perfectly comfortable, adhere to the wearing schedule; don't be tempted to wear your lenses too long too soon.

- Beware of "overwear." Halos or rainbows around lights mean you've been wearing your lenses too long. Remove them and keep them out until your vision returns to normal. This usually only takes a few hours, or overnight; if this symptom persists, call your doctor.

- Never force yourself to wear the lenses if they're *too* uncomfortable. This is no occasion for stoicism. If you find that you cannot keep up with the wearing schedule, you should maintain a shorter wearing time until that level feels comfortable; then you can gradually proceed to increase the time. If the lenses cause pain at any time, remove them and consult your doctor.

- Never insert your lenses if there is any redness or discharge; these are usually signs of allergy or infection.

- It is unwise to use an ocular decongestant (such as Visine or Murine) to "get the red out." These eye drops work by constricting the blood vessels, which further reduces the supply of oxygen. The oxygen imbalance that follows the instillation of these kinds of drops actually aggravates the problem in spite of the temporary relief. Remember, only eye drops prescribed by your doctor should be used during and/or after contact lens wear. I vividly remember one of my patients who started using an ocular decongestant once a day. Eventually he boosted the dosage to twice daily; then three times a day. He finally worked his way up to an astounding dozen times a day in order to maintain a "white" eye that appeared normal. His eyes had become so resistant to the drops that if he missed even one application, the eyes reacted by turning "beet red." It took months for me to wean him away from the eye drops. Naturally, during this period contact lens wear was out.

THE TEN COMMANDMENTS OF CONTACT LENS WEAR AND CARE

Your lenses are delicate, expensive objects. Your eyes are sensitive, irreplaceable organs. To maintain the vision, health, and comfort of your eyes and prolong the useful life of your contacts, meticulous care and handling are of extreme importance. The techniques used to insert and remove the lenses may seem difficult and awkward at first, but with time, patience, perseverance, and motivation you will master them just as thousands of others have. They'll soon become simple routines as you develop your own individual technique, and as natural and easy as brushing your teeth or tying your shoelaces. Specific procedures vary somewhat and depend upon you and the type of lens you wear. But certain general principles apply no matter what.

1. Cleanliness Is Next to Godliness. Before handling your lenses, wash your hands and face, making sure that your eyelashes are free of mascara and that the eyelids are "squeaky clean." Use a mild soap containing no creams, oils, or perfumes that may cling to your hands and cloud the lenses or cause irritation. You may want to use a special soap (Optisoap, made by Optiken International) developed especially for contact lens wearers. Use a lint-free towel to dry your hands and face. Follow the directions for cleaning, disinfecting, wetting, and/

or rinsing lenses before insertion and storage.

Don't use anything other than the specified solutions for your lenses. Don't use hard lens preparations for soft lenses and vice versa. *Do not use saliva* to clean a lens. Your mouth is full of bacteria and may cause an eye infection, to say nothing about the possibility of swallowing a lens (a bitter pill indeed). During the course of a lively dinner conversation, if your lens begins to bother you, don't nonchalantly pop it into your mouth—you may discover a bit of spinach, crepes suzette, or *Staphylococcus aureus* has found its way into your eye along with the replaced lens.

2. Set Up a Work Area. It's usually recommended that you insert and remove lenses over a flat surface covered with a clean white towel so that if a contact lens inadvertently falls it will be protected from scratches, and will be easy to find. Many people, however, find working over the bathroom sink more convenient. Just remember that such conditions are riskier if you drop a lens. *Always close and cover the drain* or be prepared to wish your lens bon voyage as it begins its travels through the city's water system.

At first you may find that sitting at a table and looking into a mirror during insertion and removal will be helpful. But you should try to break the habit as soon as possible; remember, you won't always have access to a mirror.

3. Be Gentle. Handle a lens as little as possible and as gently as possible, without pinching it between the edges. Your fingernails should be kept relatively short and smooth to avoid harming your lenses (and eyes!). Don't clean the lenses by wiping them between a tissue or cloth. A contact lens is not a pair of glasses: the delicate plastic from which they are made can be easily scratched. Routinely check your lenses for scratches and visible deposits that can affect vision and comfort and can harbor dangerous microorganisms.

4. Establish a Routine. To avoid mixing up your lenses, always work with one lens at a time, and always start with the same one (usually the *right* one).

5. Don't Be Overly Persistent. If it becomes difficult to insert, wear, or remove the lens, take a break and try again. If you still have trouble, call your doctor. If the lens becomes uncomfortable during wear, remove it and inspect it for foreign particles or deposits. It is also possible that you may have inserted the wrong lens, or inserted a soft lens inside out.

6. Remove Lenses Before Swimming, Showering, or Sleeping. Unless you are otherwise instructed, and you take special precautions, water could enter your eyes while swimming or showering. The lenses might shift, fall out, float away; soft lenses could absorb chemicals (such as chlorine) and impurities from the water. (Ask your doctor if you can swim with goggles or a mask.)

Only extended-wear contact lenses may be worn round the clock. Standard hard and soft contact lenses are worn by some people while napping, but this is not recommended since corneal swelling may occur due to a reduction of available oxygen. If you should inadvertently fall asleep while wearing standard lenses, instill a few drops of saline solution (for soft lenses) or lubricating eye drops in the eyes to loosen the lenses before attempting to remove them.

7. If You Drop a Lens, Don't Move. Look for it first; if you must move, step carefully. Enlist the aid of bystanders if possible. To pick up a dropped lens, wet the fingertip and touch it to the surface of the lens; then inspect for damage and *clean it well* before reinserting.

8. Avoid Fumes. Chemical vapors from gasoline, paint, turpentine, etc., and hair spray can irritate eyes and adhere to the lenses, especially soft lenses, causing permanent lens damage. Close your eyes for the duration that the vapors are suspended in the air, or remove your lenses if you know you'll be in such atmospheric conditions for long. If you use hair spray, spray perfume, and deodorant, allow the mist to settle fully before inserting your lenses. (Soft lenses must be replaced if damaged.) Some patients also experience discomfort in beauty shops, especially when sitting under the hair dryer, so you might want to remove your lenses when exposed to the drying effect of heat.

9. Be Careful with Makeup. Try to put makeup on *after* inserting your contacts, and remove the makeup after you've taken them out. If you find that you displace lenses frequently from the pressure, practice and a lighter touch should help, as will a change in the form of makeup used. (For instance, switch from a hard pencil eyeliner to a softer one, or to liquid. Confine eyeliner to the outer part of your upper and lower lashes; don't let it wander to the inner rims.) If you still displace the lenses, you may apply makeup before inserting them. Be sure to wash your hands thoroughly before touching the lenses; cosmetic oils and creams are difficult to remove. It's best to use water-based and hypoallergenic cosmetics such as those made by Almay and Clinique, particularly around the eyes; oil from cosmetics may remain in the eyes overnight, causing troublesome and persistent clouding of the lenses. Mascara is a frequent site of bacterial contamination; it's recommended that you replace your supply every three months whether it's depleted or not. Waterproof or lash-building types of mascara are especially dangerous because irritating specks and fibers can enter the eye and creep under the lens. I have also often been amazed at the amount of embedded mascara on the undersurface of the upper and lower eyelids. These deposits will remain forever. Though usually harmless, the deposits do sometimes act as a chronic source of infection. Any makeup containing particles of glitter is dangerous to the contact lens wearer, and can become irretrievably imbedded in soft lenses. Exercise common sense and experiment to find the procedures and types of cosmetics that best suit you—particularly the hypo-allergenic and water-soluble products.

10. Have Your Lenses Checked Every Six Months. Don't be shy about asking questions and voicing your problems during and between visits—that's what you're paying for.

It's also advisable that you carry with you at all times a card that indicates you are wearing contact lenses. In the event of an accident that renders you unconscious, the lenses should be removed so the health of your eyes isn't affected. No matter how comfortable your lenses may feel, you should keep a carrying case with you in case you need to remove your lenses in an emergency.

BLINKING

Normally, you don't think that much about blinking your eyes. Yet it's something you do between eleven and twenty times every minute. Blinking has much in common with another bodily function, breathing: both are done regularly, rhythmically, and automatically. Proper blinking is especially important for contact lens wearers since it can mean the difference between comfort and discomfort, clear vision and cloudy vision, and being a successful wearer and an unsuccessful one.

Picture your eyelids as little windshield wipers that sweep your cornea and contact lenses clean with every blink. Blinking protects your eyes from foreign particles, cleans them of any unwanted debris, provides a constant supply of fresh tears to take the place of those that have evaporated or have become oxygen depleted, and cushions the lens—in short, an important factor in your eyes adapting completely to contact lenses.

Unfortunately many new lens wearers neglect blinking frequently enough, or they don't blink correctly. With each blink your eyelids feel the lenses and shift them slightly. This sensation takes some getting used to and causes some lens wearers to inhibit the urge to blink, or to squint constantly in order to avoid blinking fully. Soft lens wearers who are sluggish blinkers may not even realize that although the eye surface underneath the lens may remain lubricated, the lens surface will become dry. You'll know if you are not blinking correctly because your doctor will spot it, or you may realize that you are suffering from any of the following symptoms: itching, redness, or a scratchy, tired, heavy feeling. A dry lens will result in blurred vision and is also more likely to pop out.

Make sure you're blinking properly by performing the following exercises after you've inserted your lenses, and every hour during lens wear. You'll soon be adapted to your lenses and blinking properly and automatically. For each blink close your eyes slowly and *completely,* bringing the upper lid down to meet the lower lid. No cheating by squinting, and no squeezing. The motion should be relaxed. Pause for a moment with your eyes closed; then let the lids open.

EXERCISE #1

Look way up to the ceiling; blink six full, deliberate, slow blinks.

EXERCISE #2

Look to the extreme right; blink six times again.

EXERCISE #3

Look to the extreme left; blink six more times.

Remember: It's the eyes, not your head, that move in all three positions.

THE COST OF CONTACT LENSES

As you know by now, quality contact lenses and quality eye care don't come cheaply. I always advise my patients not to compromise when it comes to their eyes. Cheap lenses and poor fit can prove to be expensive, especially when the lenses stay in the dresser drawer rather than on your eyes. Most important, the wrong lens or improper fit can result in damage to the eye. An educated consumer is one who knows enough about contact lenses to choose a qualified expert to fit him or her, thus avoiding discomfort, eye damage, and ripoffs. Unless the contact lenses are used to treat a disease or are used following eye surgery, they will most likely not be covered by standard medical insurance. However, save the receipts, since the lenses and solutions are tax-deductible medical expenses. It's difficult to give specific figures when dealing with contact lenses because prices vary according to the part of the country, and the quality and type of lenses. And inflation has its effect on contact lenses just as on any other consumer goods. In general, though, you can expect to pay fifty to one hundred dollars for the initial medical eye exam provided by your ophthalmologist. This is a separate entity and thus a separate fee. (This should not be confused with the brief nonmedical eye exam sometimes included in an overall fee for the "bargain" lens.) Contact lenses can cost anywhere from an all-time (and highly suspect) low of forty-five dollars per pair all the way up to six hundred dollars for special lenses. In general the standard hard lenses are the least expensive, with gas-permeable and soft lenses costing about one third to one half again as much. Extended-wear lenses, bifocal contact lenses, and special soft contact lenses that correct astigmatism are the top of the line as far as lenses go. The initial cost of the contact lens "package" includes everything you need to get started:

- *The contact lenses.*
- *A carrying case.* Used to store and carry the lenses when not in use.
- *Various contact lens solutions.* The answer to the problem of cleaning, rinsing, storing, wetting, disinfecting, and lubricating. (Varies according to lens type.)
- *A disinfection unit.* If you are disinfecting the lenses by heat, an electrical unit is used to sterilize soft lenses. You will need an adaptor if traveling abroad.
- *An accessory case.* Used to organize all the above paraphernalia.
- *An instruction session and educational information.* Personalized instruction, training films, and pamphlets describing the techniques used to insert, remove, care for, and handle the lenses.
- *Adjustments in the lenses.* Needed to improve fit and vision during the first six months of lens wear.
- *Warranty.* Lenses are guaranteed against defects (a torn lens, a scratched lens, etc.). That is why it is so important to have the lenses checked by the doctor before you wear them.
- *Office visits.* Unlimited visits to the doctor's office during the first six months to improve the fit and vision, and to facilitate the care and handling of the lenses.

Of all these items the most expensive part of the cost is the time and skills of your contact lens physician. The high-quality plastic from which the minuscule miracles are made costs only a few pennies to produce. It's the skill and workmanship, time and knowledge, that are needed to transform the plastic into a well-designed lens. More important, the expertise of the eye doctor provides you with the correct type of contact lens that allows clear vision and comfort without damage to your eyes.

(Note that a reliable contact lens practitioner will refund the cost of the lenses if, after all options are reviewed and tried, you are still unable to adapt to contacts.)

ADDITIONAL COSTS

Spare or Replacement Lens. Whether you have insurance or not, you'll have to pay for extra lenses. I advise my patients to buy a spare pair of lenses to keep handy for instant replacement.

Accessories and Solutions. Nothing lasts forever, and sooner or later you'll need a new supply. (See pp. 47–50 for an overview of contact lens solutions.)

Polishing and Cleaning. Hard lenses can have scratches and accumulations removed by polishing to prolong their useful life. This can only be provided by a laboratory and should be performed twice a year. Unfortunately no similar procedure exists for thoroughly cleaning soft lenses, which must be maintained as well as possible by the wearer on a regular basis.

Follow-up Visits. You should have a complete medical ocular examination every six months after purchasing your lenses, in order to update the lenses if necessary and to make certain that your eyes and contacts remain clear and healthy.

Insurance. This used to be an absolute necessity. Not only did people drop and damage their contacts because they weren't used to handling such delicate objects, but the hard lenses used to pop out more frequently than today's better-made, better-fitting lenses. They were also less comfortable and so more often removed, cleaned, and reinserted—and more handling increases the risk of damage and loss.

Many contact lens wearers still opt for insuring their lenses against damage or loss, but be sure to ask your practitioner for advice. Hard-lens wearers may be prone to loss, but soft-lens wearers find they must replace worn-out lenses frequently—sometimes every year. Your doctor may have an office policy or will have an established insurance policy available. Most plans are computerized to simplify paper work and speed settlements; they may be offered by insurance companies or even contact lens manufacturers themselves. Most apply a deductible like any medical insurance and usually require that you pay only a predetermined fitting fee to the practitioner who will inspect the lenses and examine the fit.

When considering an insurance plan, first find out the cost of replacing the lens without insurance. Then compare that with the cost of a lens replacement with insurance. Since the relative cost of replacing lenses has decreased over the years, it may actually be cheaper in the long run to simply buy a new lens whenever necessary, especially if you are the usual type of contact lens wearer who seldom loses or damages lenses.

CONTACT LENS SOLUTIONS

Various types of solutions are needed to keep contact lenses clean, hydrated, and compatible with the eye. The needs of soft and hard lenses differ somewhat. (Thus two sets of solutions and care systems exist—see below.) Both systems usually utilize preservatives that kill bacteria, viruses, and fungi that can cause ocular infections. These preservatives should ideally be effective against the most common of these microorganisms, but remain harmless to the eyes; at the same time, they should not interfere with the other functions of the solutions. Unfortunately no single antimicrobial agent or combination of agents that can do all that has yet been found. Substances that are capable of killing living microorganisms may be potentially harmful to the living cells in the eye. The eye sometimes becomes irritated by the very chemicals in the solutions that are supposed to protect them, and soft contact lens wearers in particular may become allergic to the two preservatives, thimerosal and chlorhexidine. (In Japan, solutions containing thimerosal have been banned.) The preservatives are not the only unsolved problem. Even with wetting solutions, hard lenses do not stay "wet" and comfortable forever; in spite of the special cleaning solutions soft lenses can't always be cleaned completely and may "wear out" by becoming "spoiled."

Your contact lens specialist will recommend specific products for you to use. It is the doctor's task to evaluate the contact lens solutions with special attention to their effect upon the lenses and upon the human eye. In this ever-evolving field, solutions are improving along with their accompanying lenses. The search for the all-in-one solution is especially keen, because this would make the maintenance process more convenient and increase patient compliance. Such solutions do exist, though in my opinion they leave something to be desired. It is better to use the more effective individual solutions for each procedure.

WHY TWO SYSTEMS?

In *hard lenses* and *gas-permeable lenses,* wetting solutions are a most important product. They are directly responsible for making the lenses more comfortable. Hard lenses have a slick, *hydrophobic* (water-hating) surface over which water and tears do not readily spread. Wetting solutions make the lens's hydrophobic surface a *hydrophilic* (water-loving) one that accepts water more readily. Wetting solutions must, however, be applied to a clean lens to be effective. So there must be a cleaning solution to remove the deposits and dirt that can accumulate during wear. A soaking and storage solution is also needed to keep the lens clean and aseptic when not being worn. Thus for hard lenses you use a system of daily cleaning, wetting, and soaking solutions.

By contrast, another problem takes precedence in *soft lenses* and *extended-wear lenses.* These are made of naturally hydrophilic plastics that are almost spongelike in their ability to absorb water. Unlike hard-lens polymers, soft lenses may also absorb other substances; thus, keeping them clean is a major priority. The traditional preservatives used in hard contact lenses will bind chemically with the soft lenses, causing damage to the lens and irritation to the eye. In addition, wetting solutions aren't necessary; however, a different procedure, disinfection, is needed. Hence soft lenses require a special system and different solutions. A daily cleaning, rinsing, and disinfection/storage system is used, along with a weekly special cleaning with an enzyme solution.

For both types of lenses there are additional lubricating products that rewet, clean, and cushion the lenses while they are worn.

Hard lens solutions should never be substituted for soft lens solutions, and vice versa! Look carefully when you buy to make certain that you get the correct solution for the specific lens.

CONTACT LENS SOLUTION INGREDIENTS

The list of exotic chemical names on the packaging is a long and puzzling one for most contact lens wearers. Here are the most important common ingredients and what they do.

Buffers. Used to adjust and prevent changes in the pH (acidity/alkalinity) of the solution to make it more compatible with the tears and the eye:

Sodium bicarbonate

Sodium phosphates

Sodium borate

Boric acid

Surfactants. Surface-active agents (detergents) that purify or cleanse:

Octylphenoxy (oxyethylene) ethanol

Polyoxyl 40 stearate

Tyloxapol

Chelating Agents. Remove metallic ions in a solution and stabilize and enhance the effectiveness of other agents:

EDTA

Edetate disodium

Disinfectants and Preservatives. Destroy or inhibit the growth of microorganisms:

Benzalkonium chloride

Chlorobutanol

Thimerosal

Phenylmercuric nitrate

Chlorhexidine gluconate

Sorbate (sorbic acid)

Wetting and/or Lubricating Agents. Cushion the lens against the eye and lubricate the lens:

Octylphenoxy (oxyethylene) ethanol

Providone

Polyvinyl alcohol

Hydroxyethyl cellulose

Polyethylene glycol 300

In addition, soft lens wearers use an *enzyme cleaner* containing *proteolytic papain,* which digests protein deposited on the lenses by tears and lid secretions.

CHAPTER THREE

STANDARD HARD CONTACT LENSES

"I can't begin to tell you how excited I was when the doctor put in my contacts for the first time. A whole new world opened up for me—finally I could see what I really looked like. A miracle, because I hadn't seen myself without glasses for as long as I could remember. I was the classic four-eyes: the studious, introverted, myopic kid . . . always 'losing' my specs because I hated them so. I was really unpopular in high school; by then my lenses resembled Coke bottles. I only wore the despised spectacles when I *had* to, which meant I never said hello to anybody. How could I? I couldn't *see* them! But I kept squinting through life, convinced that the only two people who belonged in glasses were Phil Silvers and Woody Allen. Then a friend of mine got a pair of contact lenses. She looked great; she loved them; I decided to join her. That was literally the beginning of a whole new life for me. I admit I had a hard time adjusting; but I wanted to be free of glasses more than anything in the world, so I stuck to it. It was worth it. My new appearance gave me the impetus to go on a diet, no less, and to come out of my shy, retiring shell. Now it's sixteen years later and I still get a thrill when people tell me 'What beautiful eyes you have.' I can't imagine ever living without contacts."

The standard hard lens is the grandfather of all the modern contact lenses. It's still quite popular, but advancements in the other types of contacts have caused hard-lens use to decline at a rate of 10 to 15 percent each year. Hard (or, to use more pleasant terms, "rigid" or "firm") contact lenses are small, firm, plastic discs that rest on the cornea of the eye, cushioned by a layer of tears. The plastic from which conventional hard lenses are made is called *PMMA* (polymethyl methacrylate) and is similar to Lucite and Plexiglas. PMMA has an excellent optical quality and has been proven to be nontoxic, stable, and highly resistant to warpage.

Hard contact lenses are, relatively speaking, "old hat" by now. There are dozens and dozens of manufacturers who, by and large, offer the same product. Unlike soft lenses, hard lenses do not require the rigorous testing and Food and Drug Administration approval before they can be legally dispensed. "First quality" hard contact lenses merely have to follow the voluntary standards set up by the American National Standards Institute. Based on information gathered over several decades of hard contact lens use, these standards apply to the following lens properties: hardness, strength, flexibility, scratch resistance, resistance to impact, absorption of saline and distilled water, gas permeability, wetting angle, light transmission, heat distortion, and shelf life.

WHO SHOULD WEAR HARD LENSES

Though many factors should be considered during the discussion between you and your contact lens specialist, generally, hard lenses will be the lens of choice if you:

- Must have the sharpest visual acuity possible.
- Have a high amount of astigmatism.
- Have moderately "dry eyes."
- Are concerned about the cost.
- Use topical eye medications.
- Prefer an easy lens care system.
- Desire a durable lens.

NEW DEVELOPMENTS IN COMFORT

One of the reasons for rigid-lens failures is due to the fact that PMMA allows neither oxygen-rich air nor oxygen-rich tears to pass through it. Your cornea needs oxygen to remain healthy; in hard lenses it relies mainly on the tears that flow under the lens and are replenished with each blink. If the tears' supply of oxygen isn't sufficient, the lens is uncomfortable and can't be worn for very long. (Gas-permeable contact lenses, which are not made of PMMA, are a big threat to the future of conventional hard contact lenses because they retain most of the hard lens's advantages and few of their disadvantages; see Chapter Five.) Another cause of discomfort in hard lens wear is the constant rubbing of the upper lid as it crosses the inflexible lens edge during each blink. Standard lenses are being made more comfortable in several ways to overcome these discomforts.

SIZE AND THICKNESS

The modern conventional rigid lens is usually between 8 and 10 mm in diameter and doesn't cover the cornea completely. Earlier hard lenses were much larger and covered not only the cornea, but the sclera (white part of the eye) as well. Over the decades improved fitting and manufacturing techniques have allowed the lenses to gradually shrink in diameter and thickness. Now we even have "ultra-thin mini-lenses" with a center thickness of .035 mm and less than 8 mm in diameter. These contacts are very comfortable for a hard lens but difficult to fit, since they have to be centered perfectly over the pupil. Unlike the larger lenses, which have a large tolerance of movement without adversely affecting vision, these small thin lenses should move only slightly with each blink; otherwise blurred vision will occur. If a cornea is too steep or too flat or has too much astigmatism, the mini-lens should not be prescribed. For people who can wear them, however, small, thin lenses are more comfortable for several reasons. Well-fitted ones are more likely to float on a layer of tears and less likely to touch the cornea, so there's less sensation. They also touch the lids less, further increasing comfort. In addition, small lenses that are thin enough to flex during the blink help tear circulation, thereby reducing the possibility of overwear syndrome. (The larger the lens, the greater the distance tears have to travel once they've entered under the lens edge. By the time they reach the center of the cornea, much of the oxygen has been depleted.) Contacts must, however, remain large enough to cover a fully dilated pupil so that night vision isn't adversely affected. Thin mini-lenses must also be handled more carefully to avoid loss and warpage.

FENESTRATED OR VENTED LENSES

Hard contacts can be made more comfortable by drilling tiny holes or *fenestrations* through them, allowing more tears to reach the cornea. The holes are usually 0.3 mm in diameter. (Anything less than that and they become plugged with mucus; anything larger and vision is adversely affected.) They are best placed close to the center of the lens, since that is the area of the cornea that is most likely to be oxygen deprived. Because a contact lens naturally rotates on the eye, the area directly under the fenestration changes constantly, and sometimes only one hole is needed. But usually three holes are necessary.

Fenestrations are especially useful when the lens has to remain relatively large because of fitting or optical factors. They make better use of the available tears for hard-lens wearers who have a "dry eye syndrome," for inadequate blinkers, or for those wearing lenses in low humidity. There are also contacts with edged grooves or "vents" that are meant to serve the same purpose as fenestrations.

Some doctors prescribe and fit fenestrated or vented lenses routinely, especially in patients who are over thirty or who have dry eyes. They report a shortened adaptation period (with some patients wearing their contacts for eight hours the first day); decreased likelihood of overwear syndrome; and little or no spectacle blur or photophobia (light sensitivity). Others add fenestrations after normal wear has proven unsatisfactory; it's been estimated that about 20 percent of conventional hard-lens wearers will eventually need at least one fenestration. Others, however, report no greater comfort.

I have found that many patients complain of an unacceptable amount of visual distortion because of the fenestrations, or discomfort because the holes interrupt the smooth surface of the lens. Moreover, when the holes become clogged with mucus and debris, it becomes almost impossible to wear the lenses. Therefore I rarely prescribe fenestrated or vented lenses until all other possible avenues have been explored.

WETTABILITY

Another development making conventional hard contact lenses more comfortable involves reducing the *wetting angle,* which relates to the ease with which tears are able to spread over the surface of a contact lens. All surfaces vary in their "wettability": on a highly polished or waxed surface, water beads up into little balls and the angle between the surface and the droplet is very steep or high. Such a surface has a *high wetting angle.*

On the other hand, on a surface that's not waxed or polished or that's been washed with detergent, water won't form little round beads; instead it tends to flatten out and keep a low profile. The angle between the surface and the resultant puddle is very low or flat, and the surface has a *low wetting angle.*

This wettability property applies to the plastics in contact lenses. Depending on surface conditions, these plastics can vary in wetting angles. *The lower the wetting angle, the easier it is for tears to spread under the lens,* thus bringing more oxygen to the cornea. Wettable lenses are also more comfortable; putting a dry lens on your cornea is an irritating experience you'll not soon forget. Wetting the plastic lens therefore makes it easier and safer to wear. Wetting solutions were invented because water and tears will not spread adequately over an untreated, dry PMMA lens. Unfortunately the wetting solution traditionally used with hard lenses works for only about an hour. Longer-lasting methods now exist: Some lenses are more wettable because they're made of a modified PMMA; others have a lower wetting angle by virtue of a special permanent coating, and still others require constant instillation of lubricating eye drops to keep them comfortable.

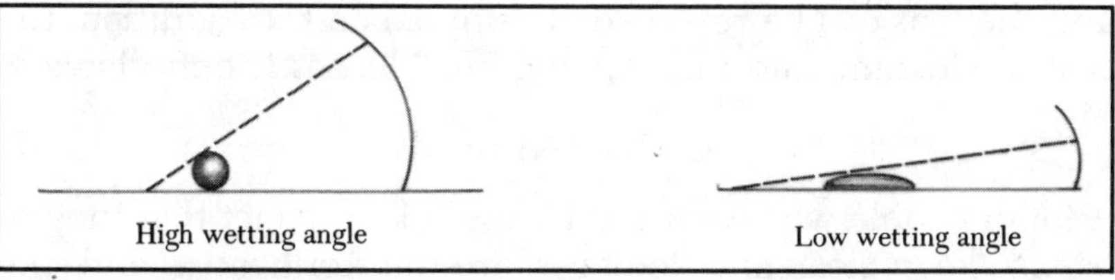

Figure 5. Wettability

ADVANTAGES OF HARD CONTACT LENSES

SHARP VISION

As many see it, the main advantage of hard lenses is that when fitted properly they provide the sharpest visual acuity for all the refractive errors—even better than spectacles can. It's not uncommon for those who have nearsightedness, farsightedness, presbyopia, and most degrees of astigmatism to report 20/10 vision—that's better than "normal"! Your prescription can be accurately ground into the front surface of a hard lens, and its smooth, firm, domelike undersurface, combined with the tears trapped beneath, forms a perfect refracting surface for the eye. A conventional soft lens, on the other hand, conforms to the shape of the cornea much like a tablecloth drapes over a table and so cannot completely correct astigmatism originating in the cornea. There are special new soft and gas-permeable lenses capable of correcting a relatively high degree of astigmatism, but hard conventional lenses are still the best for consistently correcting the higher amounts of astigmatism; besides, not everyone can deal with the soft lenses' disadvantages.

LOW COST

The next most popular plus is that standard hard lenses are the least expensive of all types of lenses. When properly handled and maintained they can last ten years and more. During that time tiny scratches and roughened edges that are bound to occur even during normal wear can be polished away at minimal cost. Also, the lens can be modified for any minor changes in prescription without ordering a new lens. Should you require a new lens, the prescription can be accurately duplicated and the lens can be replaced at minimal cost. In addition, the cost of cleaning and maintaining hard lenses is quite low.

CONVENIENCE

A lot of people who wear hard lenses like the fact that they're easy to keep clean and don't require the sterilization and special rinsing solutions that soft-lens care entails. With hard lenses all you do is rub a few drops of germicidal solution over the lens, rinse with plain tap water, and you're done. This is especially important if you're a frequent traveler who doesn't need the extra weight and bulk of several bottles of liquid sloshing around your luggage. (Not to mention the mild annoyance of a thermal disinfecting unit, which may also require a hefty electric current adaptor in some countries.) A hard lens is also easier to handle than the floppy, slippery soft lens. This is particularly true for older people. Once you have the knack, insertion and removal are a snap.

ATMOSPHERIC CONDITIONS

Since the plastic from which they are made is hydrophobic (does not absorb water), dry air doesn't affect the quality or the comfort of the lens.

COLOR

The fact that hard lenses can be tinted almost any color does more than enhance the color of your eyes. From a practical standpoint it makes them easier to retrieve when dropped, easier to locate when decentered, and reduces the light sensitivity and glare that may occur with clear hard-lens wearing. Most often hard lenses are tinted blue, gray, or green, but other tints are available.

VERSATILITY

Hard lenses have tremendous versatility. Most standard rigid lenses are *corneal lenses,* which fit over the cornea only. But *scleral lenses* exist too. These are large contact lenses that cover the white of the eye and are used for certain prosthetic and cosmetic purposes (see pp. 147–48). Fenestrated lenses, which have tiny holes drilled through them, and vented lenses, which have tiny ridges carved in the undersurface to permit a better exchange of gases, allow greater tear flow.

There are also *bifocal contact lenses.* Special corneal *cosmetic contact lenses* can be used to provide an artificial color to the eyes. They're useful for actors and actresses and others who would like to improve or intensify their eye color. The entire lens, except for the clear, central visual area, is painted or dyed until opaque. A red-tinted *X-Chrom* lens is also available, which allows the color-blind to approach near normal color perception. Another type of cosmetic contact lens is completely opaque, covers the cornea and sclera, and is used to provide a new appearance for a disfigured or damaged eye (see Special Lenses, Chapter Seven).

DISADVANTAGES OF HARD CONTACT LENSES

DISCOMFORT

Hard-lens wearers point out with a sense of irony that "they don't call them 'hard' for nothing," and suspect that the real reason their lenses are called *hard* has as much to do with the difficulty in getting used to them as with their physical rigidity. Initially a hard lens causes everyone some discomfort. (The amount varies, but at no time should you feel real *pain.* If you do feel sharp pain, either the contact lens has been improperly fitted or there's something under it.)

Hard lenses feel uncomfortable at first because, although the edges are thin and perfectly smooth, they're basically inflexible. Every time you blink, the edges of your eyelids bump against the edges of your lenses, making you very aware that the lenses are there. Ultra-thin lenses, with a central thickness of .035 mm, will flex unnoticeably a bit when you blink, and this is mostly beneficial to the tear-pumping action. You'll still feel as though there's something in your eyes (there is!), but the flexibility will allow more tears to flow beneath the lens, thus lubricating the cornea in a very effective manner.

Another source of discomfort with conventional hard lenses is that, as mentioned earlier, they're made of a plastic that allows neither gases nor moisture to pass through. For the "pumping action" to work, resulting in the vital tear exchange process, the lenses must be fitted very carefully: loose enough to allow the lenses to move slightly, but not so loose that they slip around too much and impair vision.

A by-product of the fact that hard lenses don't hug the cornea is that tiny particles of dust and dirt in a polluted atmosphere can lodge beneath the lens, causing discomfort, tearing, and redness. Your tear production may be stepped up sufficiently to banish the offending specks, but more often than not you'll have to remove the lens and clean it.

OVERWEAR AND UNDERWEAR

No matter how well your contacts fit, there's some oxygen deprivation occurring. Eventually your cornea needs a little "R and R": rest and recuperation. This varies from patient to patient, but the average time that hard lenses can be worn without removing them is about eight hours. If you overwear your lenses by exceeding your wearing schedule, your eyes will rebel and reward you with pain, redness, and blurred vision. With soft lenses signs of overwear take longer to develop. On the other hand, underwearing hard lenses by cutting down on the hours or frequency of wear tends to reverse the adaptation process; lenses should be worn the same number of hours every day. Maintenance of a constant daily wearing schedule is *essential* for the hard contact lens wearer. Intermittent wearing is definitely unacceptable.

MOLDING AND SPECTACLE BLUR

Have you ever noticed how a ring leaves a slight indentation on your finger? A hard lens temporarily molds the cornea in the same way. The amount of corneal molding depends upon the fit of the contact lens and how long it's been worn. Molding isn't harmful, but you will experience blurry vision after you've removed your contacts and put on your glasses. This is called "spectacle blur." Gradually your cornea will assume its normal shape, a process that can take anywhere from a few minutes to several hours. At that point vision with spectacles will be clear.

LOSS, SCRATCHING, CHIPPING, AND WARPING

A hard lens is more likely to pop off the eye than a soft lens. The plastic from which the lenses are made is liable to be scratched, chipped, and warped if not handled carefully. Almost every hard contact lens wearer has lived through this scenario, in a shopping center, a crowded restaurant, at a party, even in the street: She looks—too quickly—to the side. The lens pops out. She shouts *"Don't move!"* and drops to her knees. Soon she's surrounded by kneeling, groping good samaritans who've joined in the search. If she's lucky, the welcome words "I've found it!" ring out, and the lens is unchipped and unscratched. If she's not so lucky, her next move is a phone call, and later a visit, to her contact lens specialist. By the way, if you have lost or damaged one lens, you may still wear the other lens without fear of any adverse effect. Of course, you could wear eyeglasses until your new lens has arrived. I usually advise purchasing a spare pair of lenses to keep on hand in the event of just such an occurrence.

ADAPTATION TIPS

New hard-lens wearers experience varying degrees of discomfort during the initial adaptation period, which usually takes longer than for soft lenses. Follow the wearing schedule specified by your contact lens specialist (a typical one is shown below). The first few days are the hardest, and you may need a pep talk now and then to keep you on the track. During the initiation period you may experience blurry vision because of the extra tears your eyes produce in response to the foreign-body sensation. Your eyes may turn a little pink and feel scratchy. So it's a good idea to wear your lenses at home initially until your vision and appearance improve and you feel comfortable and confident enough to venture out into the real world. Establishing a good blinking habit is especially important at this stage (see pp. 43–44 for blinking exercises).

After your eye doctor is satisfied that you've been fitted with the best possible PMMA lens for you, you'll need from four to eight weeks to reach full-time wear, which is, on the average, eight hours per day. Six weeks is the average adaptation time, with the first week being the most trying.

You might at some point become discouraged and doubt that you'll ever get used to hard lenses. Although the dropout rate is very small, about half of all hard contact lens candidates that give up do so because they couldn't make it through the adaptation period. Don't let this happen to you. It is estimated less than 1 percent of the prospective contact lens wearers will not be able to adapt no matter how motivated and diligent they are, but chances are you're not one of them. Now there are so many new special lenses and improved fitting techniques that, to paraphrase one manufacturer, "there's no reason hard lenses should give you a hard time."

Millions of people have gone through the adaptation process and so can you. Every day your lenses will feel a little better; you'll be able to wear them a little longer and begin to enjoy

TYPICAL WEARING SCHEDULE—HARD CONTACT LENSES

DAY 1

Three periods of one hour each with the lenses in place. Keep the lenses off for at least one hour between each wearing period.

DAY 2

Three periods of two hours on.

DAYS 3 & 4

Three periods of two and a half hours on.

DAYS 5, 6, & 7

Three periods of three hours on.

SECOND WEEK

Two periods of five hours on each day.

THIRD WEEK

One period of six hours on each day.

FOURTH WEEK

One period of seven hours on each day.

FIFTH WEEK

One period of seven and a half hours on each day.

SIXTH WEEK

One period of eight hours on each day.

all the reasons that prompted you to switch to contacts in the first place. The byword during adaptation is "This, too, will pass." Compare it to breaking in a new pair of shoes. At first they may feel stiff or tight. But soon they become so comfortable that you actually aren't aware that you've got them on. If you're a fitness buff, compare adaptation to the beginning of your exercise program. The body protests at first and can only run one quarter of a mile or do five push-ups. Gradually you increase your capacity until you've reached your maximum or desired development. From then on it's simply a matter of maintenance. And just as a hiatus in an exercise program elicits moans and groans and a gradual buildup when you resume, so too will a break in your contact lens wearing schedule require a slow, gradual resumption in daily wearing time.

WEARING TIPS

This is a conservative, cautious wearing schedule. You may be able to wear your lenses a few hours or all day the first day, depending upon various factors: the lens type, any modifications made to increase comfort, and to some extent your eyes' physiology. You'll pay more for the new, flexible, ultra-thin mini-lenses made with wettable PMMA, but you may decide they're worth it in terms of initial and ultimate wearing time and comfort.

Always be on guard against the overwear syndrome. Once you've reached "full-time wear"—the hours will vary from person to person—you shouldn't exceed that amount. If you plan to be dancing till dawn, you should break up the wearing time. At some point during the day, remove the lenses for at least thirty minutes to let your eyes rest. Then clean, rewet, and reinsert the lenses. Your wearing time will be extended, in safety and comfort.

On the other hand, you shouldn't underwear your lenses either. Once the maximum time is reached, it is necessary to maintain that wearing schedule *every day.* If, for some reason, you do not wear the contact lenses for a day, the wearing time has to be curtailed. Reduce the wearing time two hours a day for each day the lenses are not worn. If you've merely shortened your wearing time, never wear your lenses for more than two hours longer than you did the previous day.

If only this wearer had been that cautious: "It was New Year's Eve—you know, party night. I was so excited . . . I was going with someone I really liked to the party of the year. Of course I kept my contacts on all night; crepe de chine and Annie Hall eyeglasses just don't go together. Came four A.M. and I still wasn't tired, so we stayed for breakfast. By the time I got home I'd been wearing my contacts for twenty-four hours, but they didn't hurt at all. Then came the shocker—two hours after I fell asleep I couldn't believe the stabbing pain in my eyes. They started tearing, were awfully red, and I couldn't bear the daylight. I realized this was no ordinary hangover and I called my eye doctor. Sure enough, I had corneal edema. I couldn't wear my contact lenses for three days and had to have my eyes patched for twenty-four hours. I'm fine now, but I learned my lesson; I'll never abuse my eyes that way again."

If you find your eyes are sensitive to light while wearing the lenses, you should wear sunglasses outdoors, especially in bright light. You'll need eye protection, too, when you're in windy, dusty conditions, when tiny foreign particles can get under the lenses. Wear goggles or sunglasses with side shields when you ski, snowmobile, sail, motorcycle, and so on.

Never wear hard lenses while swimming unless you wear goggles or a mask; the lenses may float away if you open your eyes underwater. Finding a contact lens in a swimming pool is probably harder than finding the proverbial needle in a haystack.

Don't wear lenses while sleeping. If you need to remove your lenses but for some reason can't put them in their storage case, there are some doctors who advise their patients to slide their lenses off the cornea and onto the sclera (white of the eye). The lenses can be left there for a long time; in fact this is routine nighttime procedure in Germany for many wearers who don't want to bother with storage and cases. I do not recommend this procedure because the lenses may strongly adhere to the sclera and it is only with difficulty that they can be removed. Also the cornea can be scratched during the sliding maneuver.

Always wash your hands before touching the lenses, and never use saliva as a wetting solution.

Never rub your eyes while wearing lenses—serious corneal injury may result.

Be sure to return to your eye practitioner for regular checkups, whether your lenses feel fine or not. He may be able to detect problems of which you are unaware, perhaps because they've crept up gradually, or simply because you may have no discernible symptoms. And, of course, do not hesitate to return for an exam if you're having any difficulties.

CARE AND HANDLING OF HARD CONTACT LENSES

Handling such small, delicate objects takes some practice. In time, as you develop your own technique, you'll be able to relax and insert, center, remove, and clean your lenses on autopilot.

Always wash and dry your hands before handling the lenses. Prepare your work area, be it sink or tabletop. Establish your routine and then stick to it to avoid mixing up the lenses. It's advised that you always start with the right lens. I place a tiny dot on the rim of the right lens of my patients to allow them to distinguish it from the left lens and to banish the right-or-left problem forever. Whenever you rinse your lenses with water, be certain the water is cool. *Never use hot water.*

HARD CONTACT LENS SOLUTIONS

Proper contact lens care includes using the proper solutions. These all play different roles in making contact lenses more comfortable and safer to wear. Essential solutions are wetting, cleaning, and soaking solutions, though you may find you occasionally need to use a lubricating solution while the lenses are in place. As is the case with the lenses themselves, the standards for hard-lens solutions are set by the American National Standards Institute. These standards apply to the solutions' functions, labeling and packaging, sterility, and the tolerance of the eye to the solutions.

Wetting Solution. Essentially, this turns a hydrophobic lens surface into a hydrophilic one that's readily kept wet by the tears. It coats the lens surface and helps prevent any bacteria and dirt on your fingertip from being transferred onto the lens during insertion. It also provides a liquid cushion between the lens and the eyelid, and the lens and the cornea, making the lens more comfortable.

Cleaning Solution. This solution removes the dirt, oil, protein, and any other residues that have built up on the lenses during normal wear. If you don't remove these particles regularly, they will collect in the micropores of the plastic, making your lenses less comfortable and less optically clear. Always rinse off the cleaning solution thoroughly with cool water and use a wetting solution before inserting a lens, because it may irritate the eye. I find that the cleaning solutions that have a gellike consistency tend to do a slightly better job than the more liquid ones; perhaps this is because they require more rubbing, an essential factor in mechanical cleaning.

Soaking Solution. In addition to further removing the oil and protein deposits, a soaking solution is a disinfectant. It protects the eye from bacterial and fungous infections. Soaking solutions also keep your lenses moist; though essentially hydrophobic, PMMA does absorb a slight amount of water. Tap water is not a suitable substitute, since the minerals it contains irritate the mucous membranes in the eye. It may also cause insoluble calcium deposits to form on the lenses, and it isn't sterile. Make certain that you change the soaking solution each day and clean the storage case with hot water once a day.

Some practitioners prefer to store the lenses in a dry state. No microorganisms except for fungus spores can survive under dry conditions.

Although both these procedures are acceptable, I prefer the soaking method and feel that the lenses are cleaner and more comfortable when kept moist continuously.

All-in-One Solutions. A few companies produce an all-purpose solution to be used for wetting, cleaning, and soaking. Although this may be a convenience, I prefer the use of separate solutions because each contains different ingredients for its specific function. Anything else represents a compromise, because the various ingredients would negate each other's effectiveness. For instance, substances that are contained in good soaking solutions negate the wetting effect; also the cleaner in a cleansing solution would be an irritant when it came into contact with the eye.

Comfort and Lubricating Solutions. These are instilled into the eye while the contact lenses are in place. They rewet, lubricate, clean, and cushion the lenses, and act as a kind of "artificial tears" that aid the spread of the normal tears. They are particularly useful for "dry eyes" that result from hormonal disturbances (such as the dryness of the mucous membranes that occurs after menopause, allergies, antihistamines, and birth control pills). They may be used as often as needed. Although the lubricating solutions are essentially the same, some patients may prefer one to another. These solutions are specially formulated to be used with contact lenses, and should not be confused with ocular decongestants, which whiten the eye and are not recommended.

INSERTING HARD CONTACT LENSES

There are several methods used to insert contact lenses. Some people use their dominant hand to insert the lenses. Others use the right hand for the right lens and the left hand for the left lens. Only practice and your doctor's advice will dictate which method is best for you.

No matter which method is used, the novice must overcome two natural reflexes while learning to insert a lens: *Looking away from the lens and closing the eyelids as the lens is inserted.* To remove a lens from the case, moisten your finger with wetting solution; touch it to the contact lens surface and the lens will adhere. After removal rinse the lens with cool tap water. Apply a few drops of *wetting solution* and massage it on the lens between index finger and thumb.

Rinse the lens again with cool tap water, inspect it to be certain that it is free of particles, reapply the wetting solution, and it's ready to be inserted using one of the methods described below. The methods describe the procedure for the right eye; simply reverse directions for the left eye.

After insertion blink several times to help the lens "settle" into place on the cornea. (NOTE: Looking into a mirror during insertion at first will help, but eventually you should learn to do without the mirror.)

METHOD #1

1. Place the contact lens with the concave (hollow) side up on the tip of the index finger of the right hand.

2. With the index finger of the left hand, raise the upper lid at its margin (base of eyelashes).

3. With the middle finger of the right hand, pull down the lower lid at its margin.

4. Fixate the vision of your right eye or look "through" the lens at all times.

5. Slowly and steadily bring your finger with the lens on it toward your eye and place the lens on the cornea.

6. Gently release the lower eyelid, then the upper eyelid.

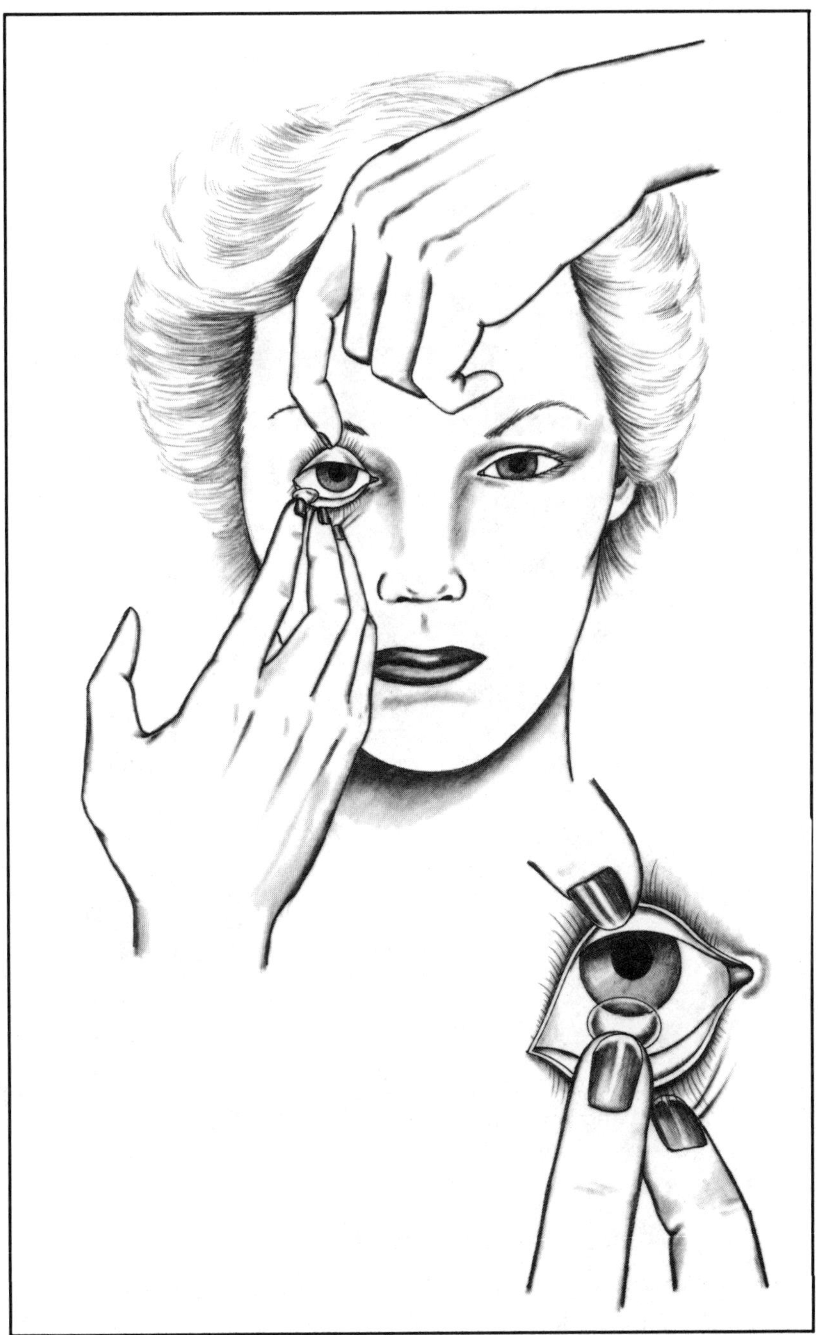

Figure 6. Inserting hard contact lens—Method #1.

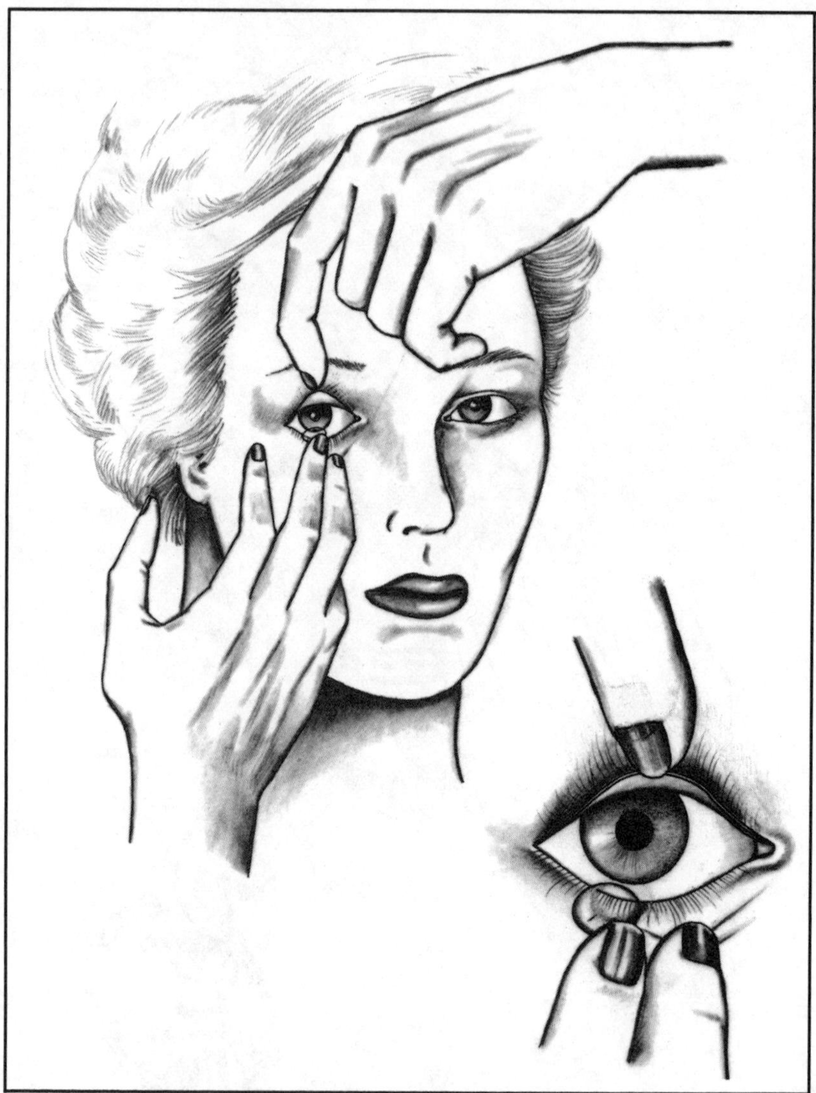

Figure 7. Inserting hard contact lens—Method #2.

METHOD #2

Same as Method #1 except that:

1. Place the lens on the tip of the middle finger of the right hand.

2. Pull the lower lid down with the fourth (ring) finger of the right hand.

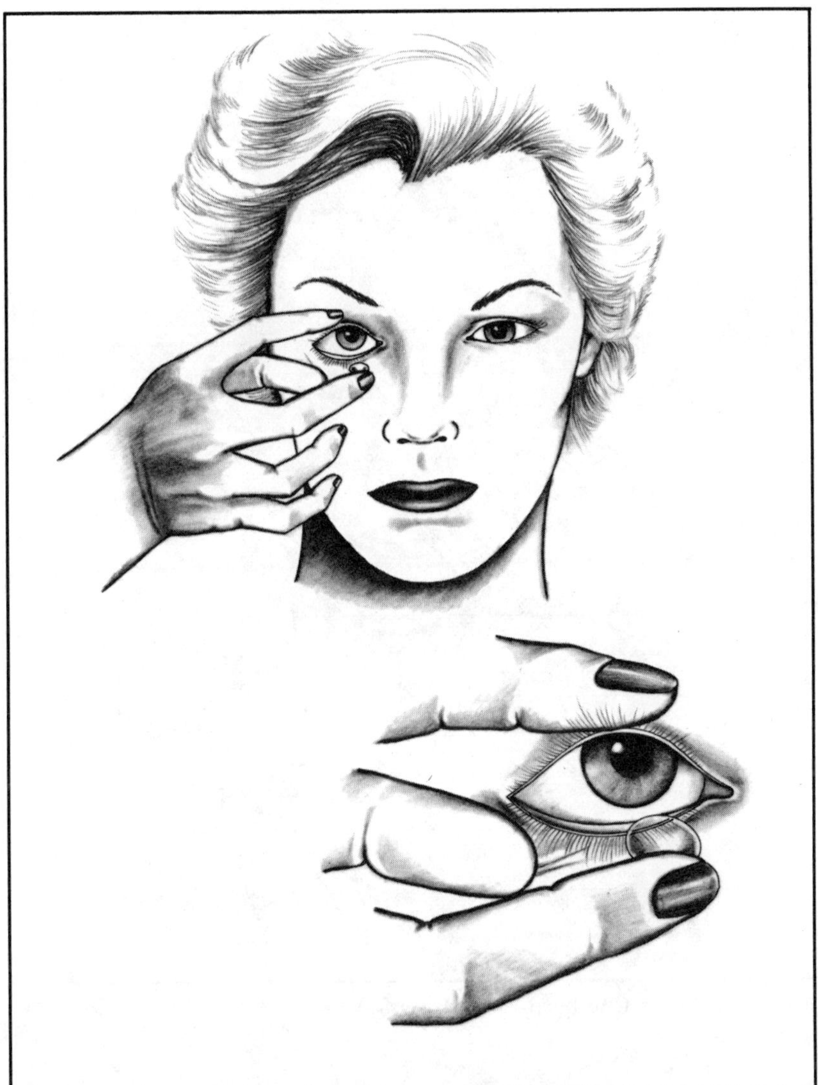

Figure 8. Inserting hard contact lens—Method #3.

METHOD #3

Use only the right hand.

1. Place the lens on the tip of the middle finger.

2. Hold up the upper lid with the index finger.

3. Use your thumb to pull down the lower lid.

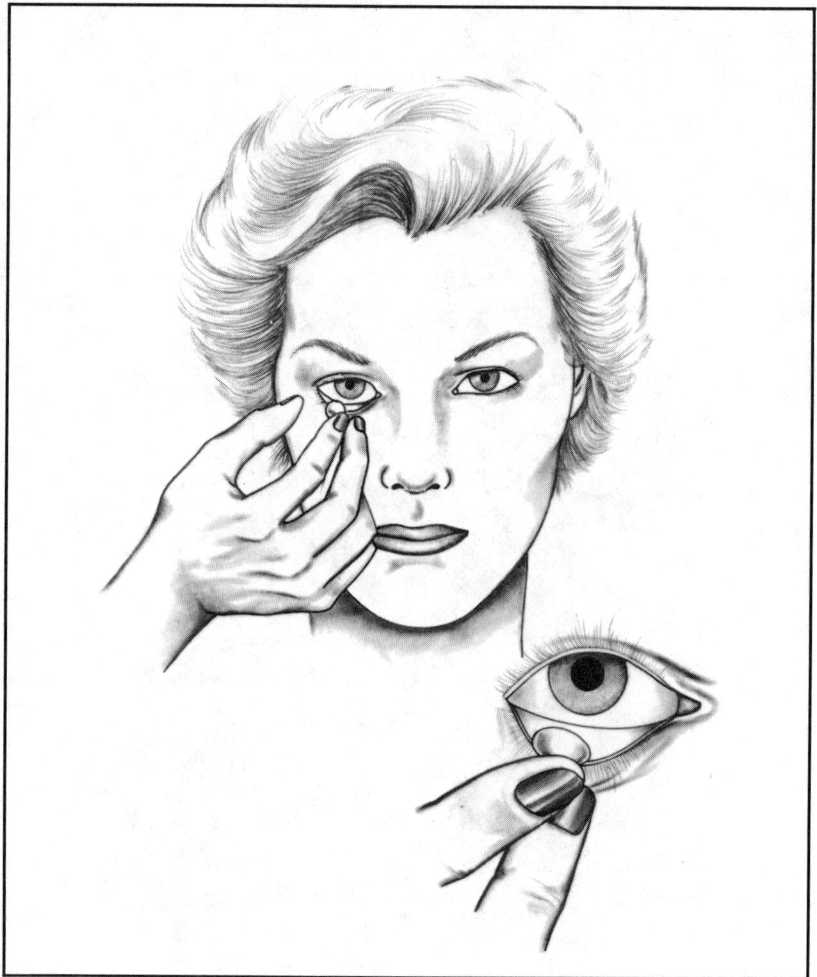

Figure 9. Inserting hard contact lens—Method #4.

METHOD #4

Again, only the right hand is used.

1. Raise the upper lid voluntarily, without help from a finger.

2. Place the contact lens on the tip of the index finger.

3. Pull the lower lid down with the middle finger.

METHOD #5

Same as Method #1 except that:
1. Place the left hand over the head.
2. Use the middle finger of the left hand to hold up the upper lid.

CENTERING HARD CONTACT LENSES

Occasionally a lens will be displaced from the cornea onto the white of the eye or under the eyelids. This may occur during wear, or during a faulty insertion. You'll know that the lens is not in place by covering the other eye: if your vision isn't sharp, then the lens is not on the cornea. Don't worry that the lens will be lost behind the eye: anatomical barriers (the conjunctiva, which covers the sclera and underside of the eyelids in a continuous sheet) prevent this from happening. Don't panic when the lens decenters; theoretically, a lens can remain decentered on the sclera for hours or even days, and there's no harm done. I remember a patient of mine who came in to have her eyes examined. A month earlier she thought she had lost a lens, and since she had a spare, she simply inserted it. When I examined her, I found her "lost" lens—on the sclera! The lens had not bothered her nor caused any damage whatsoever. So if you don't succeed at first in recentering a lens, relax and try again.

First find the contact lens either by opening the eyelids widely and looking in a mirror or feeling for the lens through the eyelid while it's closed. *Never touch the lens with your finger and push it around on the eye.* This can scratch your cornea. As with insertion there are several methods from which to choose.

METHOD #1

Look in the direction of the contact lens, and the cornea will slide beneath the lens and recenter automatically.

METHOD #2

Keeping the eyelids closed, gently exert pressure

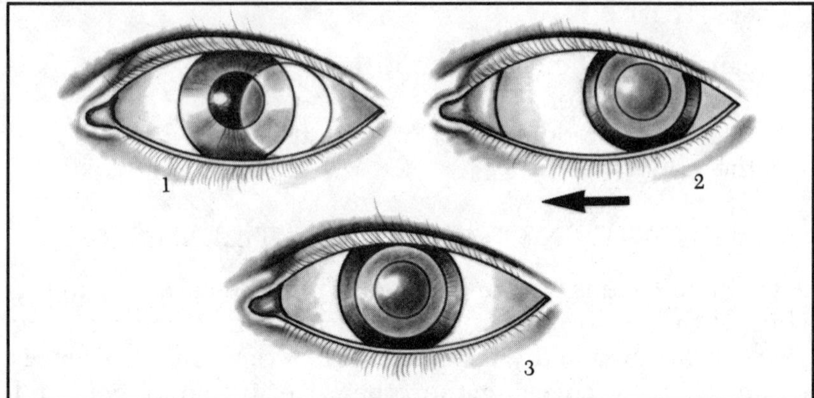

Figure 10. Centering hard contact lens—Method #1.

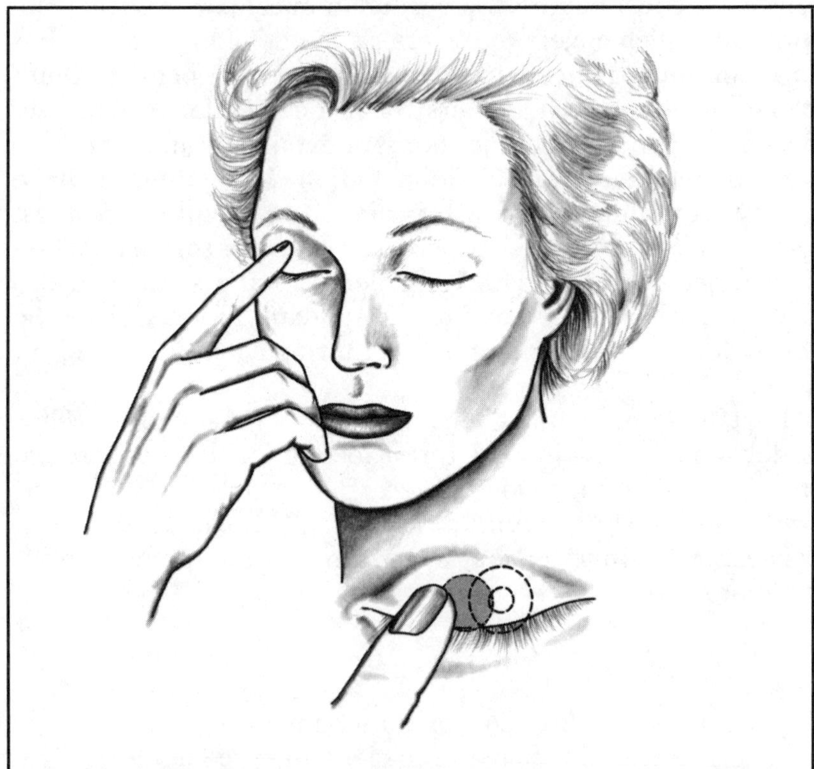

Figure 11. Centering hard contact lens—Method #2.

through the eyelids to push the lens toward the cornea with your fingers.

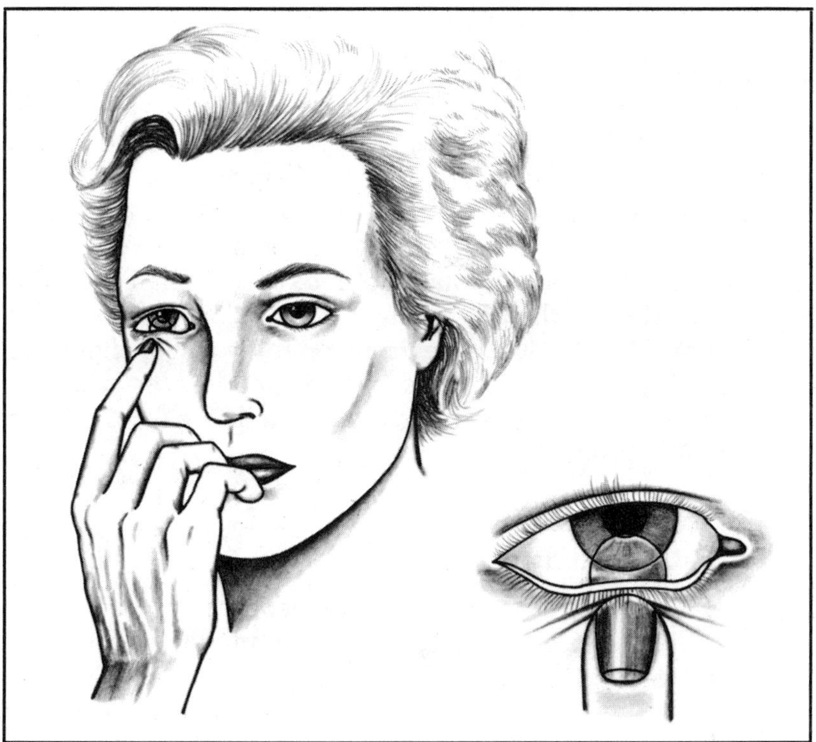

Figure 12. Centering hard contact lens—Method #3.

METHOD #3

Gently push the lens into position with the upper and/or lower lid margin. If the lens is under your lower lid, tilt your head down, look up, and use the lower lid. If it's under the upper lid, tilt your head back, look downward and use the upper lid margin. If the lens is to the side toward your ear, or in the corner toward your nose, place your fingertips on both upper and lower lids and use both lid edges to nudge the lens back in place.

METHOD #4

Sometimes the lens may adhere to the undersurface of the upper lid. In that case merely turn the upper lid inside out and remove the lens.

REMOVING HARD CONTACT LENSES

Make sure that the lens is centered properly on the cornea before attempting to remove it. Once more you have a choice of methods; your specialist will help you decide which is best for you. Always place your left hand beneath the right eye when removing the right lens and vice versa, and tuck your chin close to your chest so your face is parallel to your work surface. In all the conventional methods the mechanism is the same: The edges of the lids are forced behind the edges of the lens, to "pry" it off. Always begin by opening the eyelids very widely, as if you were surprised, so the eyelid edges clear the diameter of the lens. (The following methods are for the right eye; reverse directions for the left eye.)

METHOD #1

1. Look toward your nose.

2. Place the thumb of the right hand at the outer corner of your eye, where the upper and lower eyelids meet.

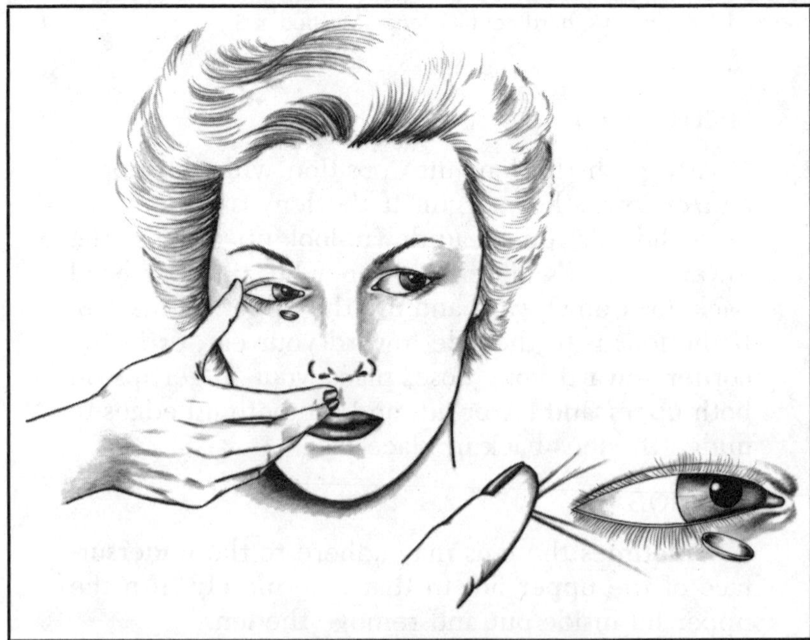

Figure 13. Removing hard contact lens—Method #1.

3. With a firm and quick motion, pull with the thumb towards the right ear, stretching the eyelids and forcing a blink. The lens will pop out.

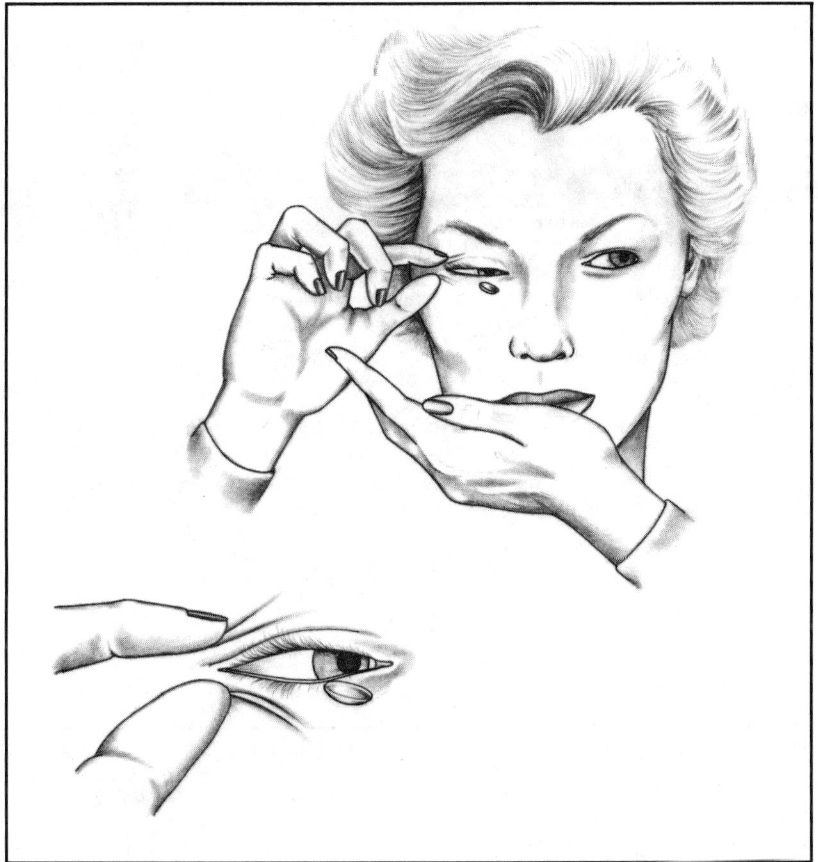

Figure 14. Removing hard contact lens—Method #2.

METHOD #2

1. Place the thumb of the right hand near the outer edge of the lower lid.

2. Place the index finger of the right hand near the outer edge of the upper lid.

3. In unison, firmly and quickly pull each lid toward the right ear and blink hard.

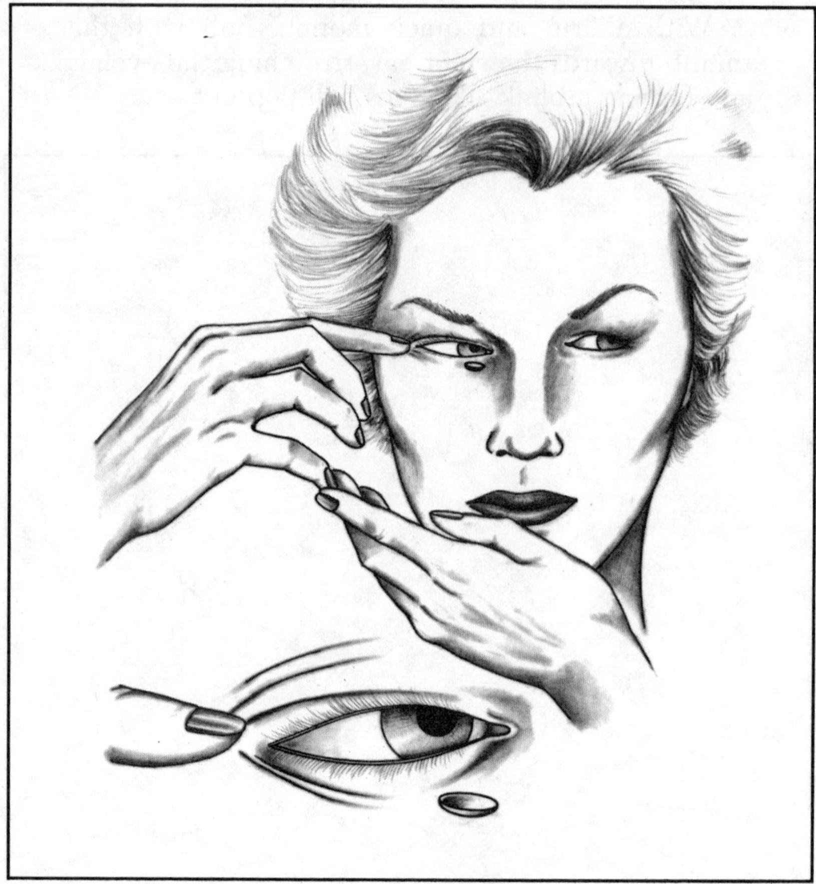

Figure 15. Removing hard contact lens—Method #3.

METHOD #3

1. Place the index finger, thumb, or middle finger of the right hand at the outer margin of the lower eyelid.

2. Firmly and quickly pull the lower lid up and out toward the right ear as you blink hard.

Alternate Methods of Removal. If all else fails, you can use either a special tiny plunger (supplied by your lens specialist), a water bath, or a touch of honey.

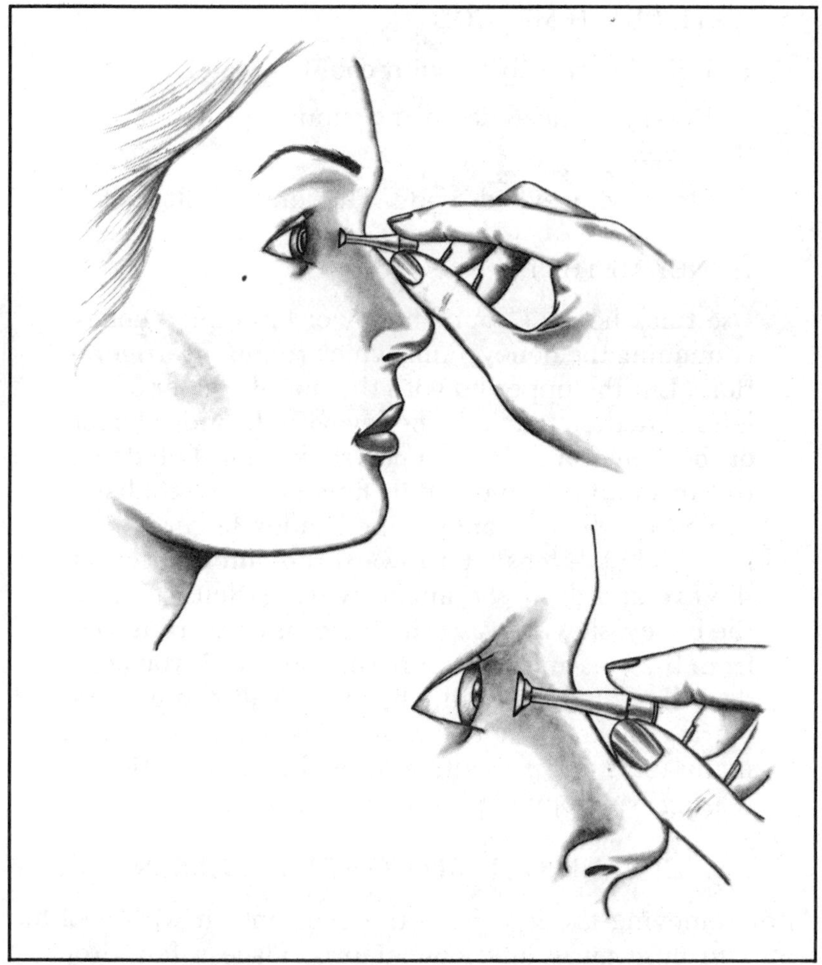

Figure 16. Removing hard contact lens—plunger method.

PLUNGER METHOD

1. Make absolutely certain that the contact lens is on the center of the cornea.

2. Look in the mirror.

3. Wet the tip of the plunger and place it lightly but firmly on the contact lens, not on the cornea.

4. Pull the plunger with the lens on it directly away from the eye. (Don't *slide* the lens off the cornea.)

WATER BATH METHOD

1. Fill a basin or bowl with cool tap water.

2. Bend your head down and submerge your face in the water.

3. Open your eyelids wide. The lens will float off.

HONEY METHOD

Use thick honey ("spun" honey or emulsified honey containing the honeycomb, which requires refrigeration). Lift the upper lid with the middle finger of the left hand, then touch the honey with the index finger of the right hand so just a dab sticks to it. Pull down the lower lid with the middle finger of the right hand as you touch the honey-tipped index finger to the lens. Slide the lens a bit toward the outer corner of the eye and draw the finger, with the lens stuck to the honey, slowly away. The honey is easily removed from the lens and will not harm your eye if you accidentally get some in it, though it will cause extra tearing. Since the honey won't stick to the lens if too many tears are present, you need to wait until the tearing has stopped if you have to try again.

CLEANING HARD CONTACT LENSES

After removing the lens from the eye, rinse it with cool tap water to flush away any loose debris. Place a few drops of cleaning solution on both lens surfaces and "massage" the lens between the thumb and forefinger or in the palm of the hand. The cleaning solution removes any residues or deposits that may have collected on the surface of the lens. Rinse the lens again with cool tap water and place it concave side up in its clean carrying case, which you have filled with soaking solution. The carrying case should be kept immaculate. Clean it every day with hot water.

In case you're wondering whether all that daily rubbing can wear out or warp and flatten your lenses—tests have proven that it doesn't. So although there are other cleaning devices that employ ultrasound waves, hydraulic pumping, and forceful sprays, you don't need them.

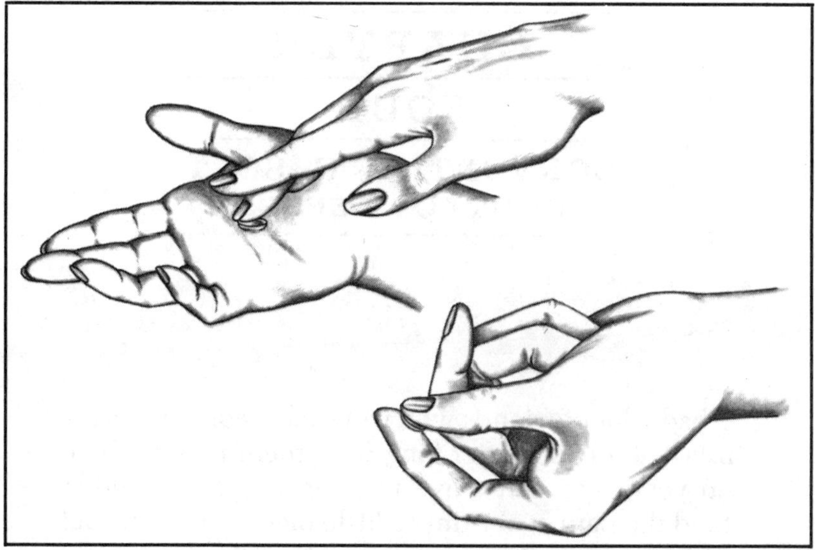

Figure 17. To clean a contact lens, massage it between thumb and forefinger or in the palm of the hand.

Some patients have resorted to using baby shampoo or liquid detergent as a cleaning solution. This is not a good idea since both these products contain alcohol. Alcohol has been shown to damage the surface of some contact lenses, causing mucus to adhere and produce blurry vision and, in some cases, a shattered lens.

STORING HARD CONTACT LENSES

Although hard lenses are made of hydrophobic plastic and won't "dry out" the way soft lenses would, I recommend that you store them in a soaking solution whenever you're not wearing them. This solution, which is mildly germicidal, keeps your lenses moist and free of bacteria and deposits. Make sure you replace last night's soaking solution with fresh solution every day. Don't try to get away with using tap water as a soaking solution. Many of the secretions from your eyes that remain deposited on your lens can combine with the minerals in tap water, and once that happens, the deposits are very hard to remove. Besides, tap water isn't sterile and won't help keep your lenses sterile either.

CHAPTER FOUR

CONVENTIONAL SOFT CONTACT LENSES

"I had a lot of friends who wore hard contact lenses; in fact, I'd had a brief fling with them myself about ten years ago. But I live in a big city and couldn't stand the pain every time a little piece of dust or soot got between my cornea and my lens. So I gave up. I don't know how my friends continued to put up with it. Actually, some of them *didn't*—gradually more and more of them began switching to the (then) new soft lenses: They seemed so happy with them. . . . They finally talked me into trying again. And, boy, am I glad they did! From the very first time I wore them they were unbelievably comfortable. I barely knew that they were there. They were so easy to wear, it was all I could to to keep myself from exceeding the hours specified in my wearing schedule. That was quite a switch from my hard-lens days, when I could hardly wait to get home to take them out. Now I wouldn't dream of going back to wearing glasses or hard contact lenses. I feel so free and I can see much better too. I'm only sorry that I waited so long."

Soft lenses' *raison d'être* can be easily summed up in one word: *comfort.* If hard lenses can be compared to a new pair of shoes, soft lenses seem to fit like an old pair of broken-in sneakers. Many wearers claim they don't feel a thing, and are completely unaware of them from the word go. Hard-lens wearers who had previously given up on these lenses are especially astounded by the lack of eye sensation because they have something with which to compare the soft lenses. No wonder more than half of all the new contact lenses that are sold are *soft*! And the percentage is increasing, although not quite as fast as a few years ago.

The soft revolution in contact lenses began over twenty years ago in Czechoslovakia, when chemist Otto Wichterle began experimenting with a plastic called *HEMA* (hydroxyethylmethylmethacrylate). HEMA had been used in surgery because of its compatibility with human tissue; it seemed to be a good candidate for contact lens material because it was also optically clear. Working in his kitchen with equipment he constructed from his children's Erector set, Wichterle concocted the first soft contact lenses. After testing was completed, more efficient and sophisticated production lines were set up. The rest, as they say, is history. The new soft lenses seemed like a cure-all—the lenses were comfortable, and in most cases the vision was good.

NEW DEVELOPMENTS IN SOFT CONTACT LENSES

The first soft lenses became available in the United States in 1971. To say there have been some changes made since then would be an understatement. The original and still highly popular Bausch & Lomb Soflens was (and still is) spun-cast of good old HEMA. But the field of soft contact lenses is a lively, dynamic, ever-changing one, with new lenses constantly coming into the market. There are now dozens of brands—numerous types of plastic whose chemical ingredients roll trippingly off the tongue (2-hydroxyethylmethacrylate, N-[1, 1-Dimethyl-3-oxobutyl]-Acrylamide and Methacrylic acid is an example). These plastics differ entirely from the synthetic material of hard contacts. Unlike PMMA, which is basically comprised of a single monomer (a substance made of low-weight molecules), soft, or hydrogel, contact lenses are made of various polymers (compounds of high molecular weight derived by combining many smaller molecules, such as monomers). These polymers, most of which are still based on HEMA, are made from a selection of at least eight different components, plus several "crosslinking" agents that bind the polymers together. The physical properties of hydrogel materials resemble living tissue more than any other class of biosynthetic material. Various methods of manufacture have also been developed, including lathe-cutting (the plastic is ground while in a hardened state) and mold-casting.

The impetus for all this ongoing activity springs from the remaining imperfections of the soft contact lens. Although a remarkable breakthrough, the soft lens is by no means a cure-all and cannot be worn by everyone. Thus the drive for improvement continues. For example, the industry is making significant headway with astigmatism and bifocals, heretofore huge flies in the ointment as far as contact lenses were concerned. The new soft *toric lenses* enable soft-lens wearers with appreciable amounts of astigmatism to see more sharply than with traditional soft lenses. (However, they still do not provide the crispness of vision that a hard lens can provide.) In the fall of 1981 soft bifocal lenses first became available to the public. For those who can't achieve normal levels of comfort, wearing time, and visual acuity with soft lenses, super-thin soft lenses may be the answer. Another improvement involves a special coating that retards the accumulation of protein deposits on the soft lens's surface, while improving the water-retentive properties. Such deposits are a major factor in shortening the life of soft contact lenses.

Surprisingly, all soft lenses are classified as drugs by the FDA because of their ability to combine chemically with medications placed in the eye. (Hard lenses do not.) The FDA must approve every new lens or lens modification as well as the solutions used in their care. Unlike hard lenses and their solutions, which have been around long enough to have been standardized, soft lenses have no established standards because the FDA insists that insufficient information still exists that would provide reasonable assurance of their safety and effectiveness. Every type of soft lens now on the market has been tested first on laboratory animals (which are "sacrificed" so their eyes can be removed and thoroughly examined), and then on a minimum of four hundred human "guinea pigs" for six months (whose eyes—thank goodness—are examined *in situ*). It costs millions of dollars and takes years to test a lens and get FDA approval. Manufacturers in this country naturally hope for a change in the required procedures, and the legal machinery for such a reclassification of soft lenses has begun to be put into motion. If soft lenses are reclassified, it would bring the cost of development down to hundreds of thousands of dollars instead of millions. It is hoped that the improvements would then come even faster, though the conservative view holds that there may still be undiscovered dangers as a result of longtime use of these lenses. (Contrast the situation in the U.S. with that of the rest of the contact lens–producing world. West Germany, Canada, and Australia—significant lens producers—are not subject to any governmental controls over their lenses or the solutions used in their care. Only Japan and England have any sort of controls, though Holland and Italy are reportedly in the midst of establishing them. Even these are nowhere near as strict as the FDA, which is looked to all over the world as the ultimate in approval. Naturally the innovations flow fast and furiously in these countries where regulation is lax or nonexistent.)

All soft lenses have one thing in common: the ability to absorb water like a sponge. This is what makes them soft and sets them apart from their firmer cousins. In the hydrated state soft lenses contain anywhere from about 30 to 80 percent water, which they get from the solutions you use and from the tears in your eyes. These water-loving lenses have the consistency of a gel, rather like firm, clear Jell-O. They're very pliable and elastic; and can be turned inside out, bent, twisted, and stretched. Yet they have a "memory" and can spring back to their original shape while maintaining the same correct prescription and fit. (This type of treatment is not recommended, however.) While they're in your eyes, soft lenses drape themselves over your cornea like a tablecloth, unlike rigid lenses, which have no such "give."

The various soft lenses differ in their water content, thickness, design, type of material, and method of manufacture. Each lens has its own set of fitting guides with certain advantages and disadvantages, and the eye practitioner must weigh all the factors carefully in relation to your eyes before deciding upon the best lens for you. You may be able to wear one type of soft lens and not another; in fact this situation is quite common. For example, the greater the ability of a lens to hold water, the better the oxygen transfer and the softer and more comfortable it may be. This type of lens will not be comfortable, however, on an eye that doesn't have a sufficient tear supply in order to keep the lens fully hydrated. Additionally, this type of lens might not provide sharp visual acuity. Soft lenses with a lower water content offer better visual acuity and usually have a longer life span, but are not quite as comfortable as those with a higher water content.

Like the hard lens, the soft lens also has its counterpart, the ultra-thin lens. Incredibly, this lens has a center thickness of less than 0.05 mm. Although they are more comfortable, these lenses are not for everyone because they are more difficult to handle and usually vision is not as clear as with the thicker standard soft lenses.

Another distinguishing variable feature of soft lenses is their size—they're considerably larger than hard lenses in order to stay centered on the cornea. From 11 to 16 mm in diameter, they are designed to fit over the cornea, the limbus (the junction between the cornea and the sclera), and part of the sclera as well.

WHO SHOULD WEAR SOFT CONTACT LENSES

The decision to fit you with soft contact lenses rests between you and your contact lens specialist. In general you're a likely candidate if you:

- Are most interested in comfort and want a contact lens that you can wear for a long period of time every day.
- Have been unsuccessful with hard contact lenses.
- Live, work, or play under conditions that are dusty and/or windy.
- Want to wear contacts intermittently, not full time.
- Are athletically inclined, especially if you water ski, snow ski, or play tennis or contact sports.
- Are not overly concerned with extremely sharp vision.
- Do not have a large amount of astigmatism.

ADVANTAGES OF SOFT CONTACT LENSES

COMFORT

Right from the start soft lenses are exceptionally comfortable, and continue to be so whether you eventually wear them all day or only part of the day. There is little or none of the rough, itchy feeling that can annoy and dampen the enthusiasm of even the most motivated hard-lens wearer. There are several reasons for this.

A soft lens has a gellike consistency, and this "forgiving" quality allows it to conform to the cornea almost perfectly. Its larger size and soft edges mean the eyelids glide smoothly over it—instead of bumping into it—during each blink. The tenacity with which it clings to the cornea prevents foreign particles such as dust in the air from slipping under the lens, a major cause of irritation for hard-lens wearers, especially in polluted areas or on windy days. Because of its clinging nature, it is also less likely to pop out.

Soft lenses are soft because they absorb water, which allows for the gas exchange that is so important to the health and comfort of the cornea. The cornea, which has no blood vessels of its own, gets its oxygen and releases its carbon dioxide directly through the air or through the tears. The soft-lens material itself is only slightly gas permeable; however, it is the tears contained *in* and *around* the plastic that allow air and carbon dioxide to pass through. Therefore more oxygen is supplied than with conventional hard lenses, which do not absorb water. A greater supply of oxygen also means that soft lenses can be commonly worn for fourteen hours or longer without harming the eye, since the overwear syndrome occurs less frequently. Though the gas exchange is better than with hard lenses, it is still below the normal rate that you find in the naked eye. Therefore it is possible for overwear to occur eventually.

Another difference between hard lenses and soft lenses is that soft lenses do not increase the eye's sensitivity to light. This reduction in photosensitivity is due to a reduction in eye irritation.

Finally, the very term *soft* is a psychological plus, and puts many a leery lens wearer at ease.

WEARING FLEXIBILITY

Soft lenses are not only physically flexible—their wearing time is flexible too. With rigid lenses you must follow a strict wearing schedule as you gradually build up to your maximum tolerance; then you have to stick to that full-time schedule daily. You can't casually skip a day or cut down a day or two without undergoing some readaptation. With soft lenses it's an entirely different story. You don't have to follow quite such a strict adaptation schedule. You'll probably be able to wear your contacts all day a week after you've gotten them.

And you can wear your lenses *intermittently* and change back to glasses whenever you want. For instance, if you wish you can wear them a few hours each day; or wear them just during the weekend and then return to a full-day wearing schedule without any adverse effect on the eye. You can even wear them for special occasions such as for playing sports or for social events without any harm to the eye.

Another factor that makes soft contact lenses fully interchangeable with glasses is that there's no corneal molding because of the plastic's softness. That means there's no annoying "spectacle blur" when you decide to wear glasses, and the oxygen deprivation and corneal edema that cause spectacle blur are less likely to occur.

SAFETY

Because of its large size, a soft contact lens acts as a "transparent bandage" that covers and protects the eye from hazards such as contact-sport injuries and foreign particles in the atmosphere.

It's extremely rare for a soft lens to pop out of the eye. No matter how rugged your sport, you can relax, confident that your lenses are safely clinging to your cornea. You can even swim while wearing soft lenses, as long as you don't dive or open your eyes too wide. The especially daring even may risk a quick dive below the surface, provided the eyes are shut tightly to prevent the lenses from floating off. I've heard of hard lenses being recovered from the bottom of a pool, but with a soft lens miracles such as this never happen. Wearing protective goggles is a good solution for those who want to see where they're swimming, but these must fit very well in order to prevent chlorinated water from seeping in and being absorbed permanently by the lens plastic. Salt water is nothing more than a strong saline solution similar to the tears and special rinsing solution you use in cleaning soft lenses. Therefore it does no harm if you accidentally get some in your eyes while swimming in the ocean. The chlorine in pool water, however, does pose a problem because of the tendency for soft lenses to absorb such chemicals. Therefore I recommend that my patients remove their lenses before entering a pool. It is advisable to irrigate the eyes with fresh water or saline solution after leaving the pool and before inserting the lenses. Snorkeling and scuba diving are possible, too—but again, the fit of the mask must be carefully made to avoid water entering the eye, possibly causing the lenses to decenter or even float off.

You can even take a short nap while wearing soft lenses, which can be a lifesaver in some situations. Overnight sleeping is completely taboo; however, catnaps with soft lenses in places do no real harm, as long as you don't make a habit of it. Your eyes might feel a bit dry and murky upon awakening, but instilling a few drops of saline solution will restore the lens and the eye to their previously compatible relationship.

DISADVANTAGES OF SOFT CONTACT LENSES

You should expect to pay about 30 to 40 percent more for soft contact lenses than for conventional hard lenses. Besides a higher initial expense for the lenses themselves, there are additional costs in the maintenance of soft lenses. For one thing they're less durable: the average life span of a soft lens is one to two years, compared with approximately ten years for a hard lens. Though relatively tough, soft lenses can tear if handled indelicately, and the lens must be replaced. They also tend to accumulate deposits from eye secretions and absorb other substances such as aerosol sprays, cigarette smoke, eye drops, makeup, creams, oils, etc. Most of these can be removed if you clean your lenses as directed, but not always. Eventually the lens clouds up, absorbs water unevenly, permits less oxygen to pass through, and must be replaced. In addition, the cleaning, rinsing, soaking, disinfecting, and enzyming solutions used to keep soft lenses in tiptop condition can add up to a sizable investment—about one hundred dollars a year. Finally, the prescription of a soft lens can't be altered in the manner of a hard lens. On the contrary, you will have to buy a whole new lens whether the prescription change is major or relatively minor. (Of course, contact lens insurance plans are available to reduce the cost of frequent replacement.)

IMPERFECT VISION CORRECTION

Soft contact lenses were once thought to be the perfect contact lens but this is not now the case. Some soft-lens wearers eventually have to switch to hard lenses or gas-permeable contact lenses. The major reason for soft-lens dropouts is the less-than-optimal vision that the lenses provide. There are several reasons for this:

Because the soft lens conforms to any irregularity of the corneal surface, the cause of astigmatism is duplicated on the outer surface of the pliable contact lens. Conventional soft contact lenses can only correct small amounts of astigmatism, and a large number of those who were fitted with soft lenses were happy with the comfort but had to settle for less-than-perfect vision. (Special soft toric lenses have since been developed, which definitely improve vision; however, they are not perfect and they cost more than conventional soft lenses. See Special Lenses, Chapter Seven.)

Soft lenses are not "custom made" the way hard lenses are, and a precise prescription can't be "carved" exactly into the surface of the lenses. A contact lens specialist has to choose from standard sizes and available prescriptions, which may result in a less-than-perfect fit for those with in-between prescriptions. And if a lens needs to be replaced, it isn't always possible to reproduce an exact duplicate of the required lens. In the latest state of the art of contact lens production, whether lathe-cut or spin-cast molded, lenses are available, like a shirt-collar size, only in certain powers, sizes, and curvatures. Also, during hydration the exact power of the lens may be altered slightly. In spite of constant checks and rechecks some lenses of inexact power may slip through. Your physician, however, should be able to detect any deviation from the prescribed power.

Visual clarity may also be erratic. During every blink the soft lens flexes, creating a moment of blurred vision. Also the constant lid pressure on the contact lens can distort the lens surface so that vision is adversely affected. (This is especially noticeable when reading. Also, when doing close-up work, one tends to blink less often and soft lenses become less hydrated than is optimal. The lens hardens slightly and reduces visual acuity.) Likewise, any change in the humidity will affect the water content of the lens, and thus its clarity. Low humidity leads to a drier, less comfortable lens and hence poorer vision.

INCONVENIENCE

Another complaint is that the care and handling of soft lenses are more complicated and time-consuming than that of hard lenses. They must not only be cleaned, they must also be disinfected daily, as a separate process. Unlike hard lenses, you can't just rinse them in tap water after cleaning. You must have a bottle of saline solution for this purpose. A once-weekly soak in a special enzyme solution is also recommended.

Travel can be a problem for soft-lens wearers. The bottles of solutions you need to carry with you are bulky and take up valuable luggage space. If you use the heat method of disinfection, you have an extra (albeit small) item to carry and there is always the problem of finding a compatible electric current. Some countries will necessitate your buying and bringing along an adaptor. There's also a special "foreign" cord, and manufacturers are experimenting with battery-operated heating units. Chemical disinfection is the alternative, but a small percentage of people will develop an allergic reaction to these solutions.

You may find soft lenses more difficult to handle than hard lenses because they're so flexible and slippery when wet, and almost invisible. Their very softness and pliability, which is so desirable in the eye, makes them more difficult to feel with your fingers. In addition, because of their size and malleability, some people find them harder to insert and remove.

NO TINT

Until 1981, tinted soft lenses were not available in this country because of lack of FDA approval. (The process of tinting soft lenses has been utilized in England since 1978.) Because the lenses are large and extend beyond the iris onto the white part of the eye, a complete dark tint would also look rather odd. But the transparency of a nontinted lens makes it difficult to see, especially when dropped. The advertising campaign based on the soft lens's near-perfect resemblance to a drop of water is no exaggeration. No tint also means no glare reduction, but since photosensitivity in soft-lens wearers is relatively rare, this is a minor disadvantage.

However, this ban may no longer be an issue for soft-lens wearers, because in June of 1981 a tinting process for soft lenses was made available. The physician may send any FDA approved soft contact lens to a special laboratory in North Carolina in order to be tinted according to certain specifications. A 1.5 mm border and a 4 mm diameter central zone are left clear in order for the lens to appear normal on the eye and to correspond to the pupil. The remaining "iris" area is then tinted, using a special process that permanently bonds the color to the lens. Because the inner surface of the lens, that part that comes in contact with the cornea, remains free of the tint, the process is in compliance with the FDA regulations. In addition, the color is safe, will not leach out, and holds up under either chemical or heat sterilization. Any color (blue, green, brown, etc.) may be specified, in intensities varying from 10 to 30 percent. Later that year Ciba Vision Care obtained FDA approval for their light blue Softint™ lens. Tinted soft lenses may become the rule rather than the exception.

DRY EYES AND AIR

Those people with inadequate tear production are poor candidates for contact lenses in general, but especially for soft lenses. The drier the eye, the harder the lens should be; therefore someone with moderately dry eyes may be able to wear hard lenses successfully, but not soft. When a soft lens dehydrates in the eye, the edges may harden and curl away from the cornea, causing discomfort and possible lens fallout. Anywhere the air is dry—the desert, an airplane, an air-conditioned or heated home or office—will adversely affect hydration and thus the comfort of the lens. One of my patients kept returning to my office complaining of red, itchy eyes and frequent popping out of his soft lenses. I finally determined that the office in which he worked had an extremely efficient air-conditioning system and consequently the air was very dry. I couldn't change his job, but I did recommend he try two procedures: that he blink more frequently, and that he instill lubricating eye drops frequently during the day. Both these procedures combined to solve his problem. During air travel the low humidity within the airplane may cause you discomfort, in which case you can simply remove your lenses and switch to eyeglasses.

ADAPTATION AND WEARING TIPS

In general you should follow the same adaptation and wearing suggestions given for hard contact lenses (pp. 60–63). However, there are a few exceptions:

Soft lenses require very little adaptation time in comparison with hard lenses. This does not mean you should treat the wearing schedule your doctor gives you casually. (A typical schedule is shown on p. 92.) Be consistent and follow the wearing schedule during the initial period. Since the contacts are so comfortable, you may not even feel them and may be tempted to exceed the recommended hours. This is not a good idea, since your corneas still need to adapt to the presence of a foreign object, no matter how comfortable it feels. Soft lenses can still be overworn, which leads to problems with the cornea such as oxygen deprivation and edema (swelling).

After you've gone through the initial adaptation period, intermittent wear is perfectly acceptable. You don't have to follow the full-time everyday wear that's mandatory with hard lenses. If you don't feel like wearing them for a day or two, or want to cut down the number of hours, it's no problem. However, if you cease wearing them completely for a number of weeks and then decide to go back to full-time wear, I suggest that you only wear your lenses for five hours the first day and gradually build up again to all-day wear. It's necessary to disinfect the lenses before inserting them again.

TYPICAL WEARING SCHEDULE—SOFT CONTACT LENSES

DAY 1

Three periods of two hours on.

DAY 2

Three periods of three hours on.

DAY 3

Three periods of four hours on.

DAY 4

Two periods of five hours on.

DAY 5

Two periods of six hours on.

DAY 6

Ten hours on.

DAY 7

Twelve hours on.

DAY 8

Thirteen hours on.

Since a good tear flow is so very important for soft contact lens wearers, make sure you practice the blinking exercises shown on pages 43–44.

The amount of lens sensation varies from person to person according to the individual's threshold of pain tolerance. You may feel as though there's something in the eye initially, but this passes as your eye adapts. If the sensation persists, remove the lens, clean it, rinse it, examine it, and reinsert it. There may have been a foreign particle under the lens, or the lens may have been inside out. If, after these procedures, the irritation persists, have the lens and your eyes checked by your doctor.

After Day 8, one hour is usually added each day until the wearer has reached his or her own maximum wearing time.

CARE AND HANDLING OF SOFT CONTACT LENSES

Soft contact lenses must be handled very carefully since they can easily tear. Handling, inserting, centering, and removing soft lenses will soon become second nature and you'll rapidly find your own efficient style and technique.

Wash and dry your hands thoroughly before touching the lenses. Not only are creams, oils, makeup, and so on a danger, but the minute amount of proteins on your unwashed fingertips can inactivate the preservatives in the contact lens solutions, so strict hygiene is a must. Prepare your work area before you begin and acquire the habit of always starting with the right lens first so you lessen the chances of a lens mixup.

Because of the nature of the plastic from which they are made, it's especially important that you remember to keep soft lenses constantly hydrated. When they're not in your eyes, they must be kept in a sterile saline solution. A dried-out lens becomes very brittle. Therefore handle it gingerly and rehydrate it by soaking it in a saline solution.

SOFT CONTACT LENS SOLUTIONS

Hygiene is of the utmost importance when handling and maintaining contact lenses, especially soft contacts. Both cleaning and disinfecting must be done every time you remove your lenses. Cleaning removes surface deposits and is performed with a surfactant cleaning solution. Disinfection kills microorganisms and is accomplished either with heat and a *saline solution* or with a chemical (cold) *disinfecting solution.* A third process utilizes *enzymes* to remove stubborn protein deposits and is usually needed once a week. Saline solution is used to remove the other solutions from the lenses. Finally, although soft lenses are quite comfortable, some wearers may occasionally find a lubricating solution or drops helpful. (The use of these individual solutions is explained below.)

Like the lenses themselves, the products used in conjunction with them must be tested before they are approved by the FDA for the general market. The contact lens manufacturer and your practitioner may recommend a specific system based upon the chemical composition of the lenses and the way they react with your own physiological makeup. Particular brands do have their die-hard fans who swear by their products and complain of problems when they switch to another brand. Should you develop an allergic reaction or sensitivity to one of the ingredients in a particular solution, you'll need to switch to a brand that omits the offending agent. The preservatives most often implicated as causing such reactions are *thimerosal,* a mercuric compound, and *chlorhexidine,* an active ingredient in certain surgical soaps.

Above all, though, never use the solutions formulated for hard contact lenses since those hard-lens chemicals will be absorbed by the soft lens and will permanently ruin them. Don't be tempted to experiment on your own. Make sure you read the label carefully before buying and listen to the advice of your contact lens specialist. Even if you have the correct soaking, cleaning, and rinsing solutions, there's the possibility of mistaking one for another. For instance, you might inadvertently rinse the lens with cleaning or soaking solution. On a short-term basis this will not cause permanent damage to the lenses or to the eye. However, over a prolonged period of time the lenses will deteriorate and the eyes can become irritated.

SALINE SOLUTIONS

Saline solution (0.9 percent sodium chloride) is the common thread that runs through the soft-lens maintenance routine. After using any of the other solutions—cleaning, chemical disinfecting, or enzyme—soft lenses should be thoroughly rinsed with saline to flush away all traces of dust, dirt, deposits, and the solutions themselves, which contain chemicals that could prove very irritating to the eyes. If you use the thermal disinfection ("heat") system, after cleaning, the lenses should be immersed in saline to keep them hydrated during the process. (Saline solution is, by the way, the basic component of many other contact lens solutions to which special agents are added.) Saline is also the last thing that should come into contact with soft lenses before insertion, and may be compared with the wetting solutions used in hard lenses, which make the lenses compatible with the eye. Saline solution can even be used alone to clean the lenses in some cases.

Today there is an array of forms and brands of saline solutions that can easily confuse the consumer. Basically they're all designed to mimic the salt composition of the tears in your eyes. Ideally they should be pure and devoid of harmful chemicals that can be absorbed by the indiscriminate soft-lens plastic. They should also be sterile to avoid introducing harmful microorganisms to the eye. It's these last two criteria that are the most difficult to meet.

There exists a controversy among physicians as to which type of saline solution to use. Each type has its advantages and disadvantages, as you will see. The main point to remember is that whatever solution you use, make certain that you follow the instructions of your physician to the letter.

Salt Tablets. In the beginning (1971), there was the salt tablet. With one 250 mm sodium chloride tablet mixed with one ounce of distilled water, contact lens wearers could make their own small batches of saline as needed, and at a minimal cost. The result was salt and water, pure and simple. However, in October 1978 the FDA voiced its concern that the homemade solution posed a hazard to consumers because of a number of factors: poor patient compliance, the potential for faulty mixing and measuring, and possible microbial contamination. I had one patient, for example, who thought that if one salt tablet was good, two were better. At the other end of the spectrum there were those patients who used only half a tablet in an attempt to stretch the solution. Still others refrigerated their saline solutions so they'd keep longer; they intended to save money and reduce the frequency of making the saline solution each day by this cumbersome method. As a result salt tablets (made at the time by Bausch & Lomb and Blairex) were taken off the market, leaving available only the sterile, premixed preserved saline solution that had received FDA approval.

Several manufacturers eventually entered the preserved saline market. However, a small percentage of patients became allergic to the preservatives used in the saline. Therefore the pendulum has swung back to a preference for unpreserved saline, available since July 1980 in either the reinstated, FDA-approved salt tablets or the premixed, sterile unit packs discussed below.

Few people may realize that salt tablets are now back on the market, especially the newcomers to soft contact lens wear. Because of the possible dangers of misuse and contamination, it is recommended that if you use salt tablets, you take the following precautions: Always mix a fresh batch of saline every day; avoid using yesterday's solution for rinsing and disinfecting the lenses or for rehydrating them while in your eyes. Use only U.S.P. salt tablets (others, such as those for heat prostration, contain added chemicals). Mix them with distilled or purified water that is also labeled U.S.P. (United States Pharmacopeia), purchased in drugstores. Steam-distilled water is best; chemically distilled water and other bottled waters (such as spring water) contain substances that could be absorbed by the lenses. (I recommend keeping the bottle of water in the refrigerator to reduce the chance of bacterial contamination.) Use the approved plastic bottle that comes with the salt-tablet kit to mix the saline, and be sure to add the correct amount of distilled water as indicated by the fill line on the bottle. The tablet takes about fifteen minutes when left to dissolve on its own. If you're in a hurry (as you probably will be if you mix it up fresh every morning), shaking the bottle speeds up the process considerably. Once dissolved, the saline is ready to use for cleaning, rinsing, or sterilization purposes, within the next twenty-four hours. Once a day clean the plastic mixing bottle very well by flushing it out with hot tap water.

Premixed Preserved Saline Solution. These contain just the right proportion of salt, plus preservatives (such as thimerosol, chlorhexidine, or sorbic acid) to ensure that the solution stays sterile, plus buffers so the pH (acid balance) more closely resembles that of human tears. All well and good, except these solutions cost more than homemade saline, and some users become allergic (eyes become red or itchy) to the preservatives. When this form of saline was the only one available, many members of the captive audience protested—and rightly so—that this "cure" was worse than the "disease" it sought to cure. (Especially since the preserved solutions merely reduce the chance of eye infection, but don't eliminate it completely.)

It is obvious, though, that preserved saline minimizes the possibility of patient error and is more convenient (there's nothing to mix). It definitely inhibits the growth of bacteria and fungi, so there's no need to replace it with a fresh batch every day. I have found that approximately 20 percent of my patients eventually become allergic to the preservatives in this type of saline, but for the remaining 80 percent preserved saline is highly effective and has no side effects. If a patient should develop an allergic reaction, I merely switch him to the unpreserved solution.

Premixed Unpreserved Saline Solution. To solve the dilemmas posed by the other two forms, a third type of saline now exists. Sterile, premixed, preservative-free saline in vials or packets is available to satisfy the cautious and/or sensitive few who can't tolerate the preservatives but who like the convenience and want to reduce the risk of possible bacterial contamination. Unfortunately, saline in this form must necessarily be packaged in small, individual doses to be opened, used, and discarded daily. (Once opened the packets are no longer sterile, the way Band-Aids are contaminated upon opening, but can safely be used for up to twenty-four hours.) That makes this form even more expensive than the preserved solutions—and it is not as widely available. The small packets, however, travel well to the office, or farther from home. On trips you can transport the exact amount of saline you need, and discard the empty packets as you go along.

Using Saline Solution. To clean the lens with preserved or unpreserved saline, a simple method is to place the lens in the palm of the hand and fill the cupped palm with saline. Rub each side with the index finger of the other hand for twenty to thirty seconds. Then rinse with more saline. (For more information see "Mechanical Cleaning," pp. 103–4.)

To rinse the lens with saline after cleaning, disinfecting, or enzyming, place the lens in the palm of the hand or hold it between index finger and thumb. Direct a steady stream of the solution at the lens using either the entire packet or equivalent (about one ounce) for both lenses. Be generous with the saline; this is not the place to skimp. Rinsing will remove potentially harmful agents that could adversely affect your lenses and your eyes. After heat sterilization the lenses may be kept stored in the case in which they were sterilized, covered with saline solution, until you're ready to insert them. As a precaution, you should disinfect the lenses if you've left them in saline for more than a few days.

A lens with embedded deposits will be uncomfortable, less

pliable, permit less oxygen to pass through, and result in reduced visual acuity. If stubborn deposits cannot be removed with the conventional cleaning and enzyme methods, I recommend that my patients use either fine table salt or baking soda along with saline solution. Put a few drops of saline in the palm and add a pinch of the salt or soda. Place the dirty lens in the salt bath and rub gently with the index finger of the other hand for a few minutes. You can safely perform this cleaning method once a week if needed. Admittedly this is a last-ditch effort; the method may prove fruitless and a new lens may have to be ordered.

CLEANING SOLUTIONS

The very characteristic that makes soft lenses so comfortable —their ability to absorb moisture—is a two-sided coin. Unfortunately soft lenses will also absorb just about everything else they come into contact with, including cigarette smoke, deposits from your own tears, makeup, and aerosol sprays such as deodorants, room fresheners, hair sprays, etc. If these deposits are not removed daily, when still "fresh," they may harden and lead to cloudy, damaged lenses that will be uncomfortable and unable to correct your visual defect properly. Lenses badly cared for will need to be replaced more often than those that are kept scrupulously clean. I often see patients in my office with "spoiled" soft lenses—full of deposits that they failed to remove, marred by pits and cracks, or tainted with bacteria. Once deposits have taken hold, they become embedded in the lens material; even if they could be removed, the lens would be left pitted.

Special soft-lens surfactant cleaning solutions are meant (but not guaranteed) to remove surface deposits. In addition to detergents they contain preservatives to inhibit the growth of microorganisms, and cushioning agents that keep the lens from becoming damaged during the rubbing. In all cases the mechanical rubbing plays a very important role in the effectiveness of a surfactant cleaner.

To use the cleaning solution, apply a few drops to each surface of the lens and either rub between your index finger and thumb or massage in the palm of your hand with the index finger of the other hand (See figure 17 on page 79). Rub each side for at least twenty seconds, making sure you clean the outer edges as well as the center. Make sure the lens is well hydrated before applying the cleaning solution. Always rinse off the cleaning solution thoroughly with saline because it can leave a film that will eventually cloud the lens, especially if you use thermal disinfection afterward. Any deposits or impurities on the lens can be permanently baked into it by the heat method. Therefore it is imperative that the lens be absolutely clean before heating. Studies have also shown that a dirty lens absorbs more preservatives than a clean lens, another reason for thorough lens cleaning before storage and disinfection.

DISINFECTING AND STERILIZING

In addition to deposits, soft lenses can carry and introduce microorganisms to the eye. This can then lead to infections, which preclude lens wear until they are cleared up. More important, infections can lead to complications if left untreated. Using a surfactant cleaner removes some organisms, but it cannot remove them all. Those that are left behind, it is feared, may find the soft, water-containing plastic a highly desirable breeding ground. Hence the need for disinfection to kill the remaining bacteria. (Lest you become unduly alarmed: The eyes have their own natural form of protection—tear immunoglobulins and the enzyme lysozyme—that combats infection up to a point. Also, soft-lens wearers who clean and disinfect their lenses as directed suffer no higher incidence of infection than either hard-lens wearers or those who wear no contact lenses at all.)

There are two methods of disinfection used to keep soft contact lenses free of organisms that could lead to eye infections: *chemical* (cold) disinfection and *thermal* (heat) disinfection. Which one you choose to employ depends upon several factors; each method has its own advantages and disadvantages. No matter which you elect, the process is an adjunct to —not a substitute for—the daily cleaning and weekly enzyming process. Disinfection must be done every day to finish the job that surface cleaning has begun. (It's not necessary, or even desirable, to disinfect more often than once a day. If you remove your lenses during the day and intend to reinsert them, simply clean them and then store them in sterile saline until you're ready to reinsert them.)

It's not recommended that you switch back and forth between the two methods because the boiling process can cause the chemicals that are absorbed by the lenses during cold disinfection to turn the lenses cloudy. Some patients do alternate methods and report no ill effects thus far. However, to perform the switch safely it is recommended that you first clean the lenses thoroughly with a surfactant cleanser and rinse with saline. Then *leach* the chemicals from the lenses. This purging process is accomplished by soaking the lenses, in their case, in a saline "bath" for two to three hours. Repeat the baths at least three times, changing the saline each time. Then you can proceed to sterilize them. Some experts advocate using plain distilled water instead of the saline for the purging, but using saline for the final bath. Shaking the soaking case speeds the process, and using a device called Swirl Clean™ is even faster.

Chemical sterilization is more popular in other parts of the world, but in the U.S. the heat method is preferred for a number of reasons: although it doesn't kill all forms of microorganisms, it destroys a wider range of bacteria than does chemical disinfection. It has a longer track record than the cold method. There are no allergic reactions, especially if unpreserved saline is used. And with the new small heat units it is convenient and just as easy as the chemical method. (As one soft-lens wearer who opted for thermal sterilization said: "I figured that the fewer chemicals which came in contact with my eyes, the better.")

Chemical (Cold) Disinfection. There are several disinfection solutions on the market. Disinfection solutions contain chemicals such as thimerosal and chlorhexidine in sufficient concentration to kill the most common microorganisms. Since the lenses remain in the solution for long periods of time, they are kept wet and free of deposits.

The cold disinfection process is simple, and only slightly more inconvenient than storing hard contact lenses. After cleaning and rinsing the contact lenses with saline, they are placed in a special storage/disinfection case, covered with the disinfection solution and left for at least four hours, usually overnight. Make certain that the storage case is rinsed daily with hot tap water and that it is free of any impurities before use. The lenses are then rinsed again with saline before insertion. Because of its relative convenience and simplicity, many contact lens wearers prefer this method over thermal sterilization, especially those who travel frequently. Unfortunately, the soft-lens plastic absorbs a certain amount of the preservatives contained in the solution, and after a while the wearer may develop an allergy to the chemicals. Approximately one fifth of those who start out with chemical disinfection will eventually change to heat disinfection because of this allergic reaction.

On the horizon are different disinfecting systems that don't contain the two preservatives named above. One utilizes hydrogen peroxide, a system that has been used by doctors in this country, and outside the U.S. by consumers for years. Another utilizes sorbate, or sorbic acid, and is now available in the U.S.

Thermal (Heat) Disinfection. A safe, effective alternative to cold disinfection is heat, which will also destroy harmful bacteria. After lenses are cleaned and rinsed with saline, they are placed in a special case containing saline solution. The case is placed in the thermal unit, which heats up after you switch it on. In older units there is a well into which you pour distilled water. When this water has boiled away, the lenses are sterile. Newer units utilize dry heat. The unit shuts off automatically, and most people sterilize their lenses before going to bed and let them stay in the unit overnight. The process actually takes less than an hour, including the time required for the lenses to cool before they can be reinserted. The problem with heat sterilization is that many wearers find it a nuisance. In addition, incomplete cleansing and rinsing of the lenses before sterilization may cause deposits to be baked into the lens surface. This method is also tougher on the plastic and may shorten the life of the lenses. There are certain lenses (such as the extended-wear lenses, Perma-Lens, Hydrocurve, and Sauflon) that hold up particularly badly under high heat sterilization. You should consider investing in a newer "dry," "low" heat thermal unit if you've been using an older model. The newer models are smaller, function with a lower but equally effective temperature, and are easier on the lenses. Also, you needn't put distilled water into the lower chamber, thus adding to the convenience.

Occasionally a heating unit will malfunction by failing to

turn off, turning off soo soon, or not turning on at all. Though a nuisance, this is no cause for panic. As an alternative you can place the lenses in their carrying case in a pan of boiling water for thirty minutes. Remove the case from the pan and let the saline and lenses cool to complete the process. This method may also be used when traveling if you forget or decide not to bring your heating unit with you.

ENZYME TABLETS

Cleaning with a surfactant cleansing solution and disinfecting may not remove all the deposits that cling stubbornly to the lens surface. To remove these deposits a special enzyme solution is used; this "digests" and dissolves lens proteins much the same way the enzymes in your body help break down protein.

You should use the enzyme cleaner once a week to help prevent buildup of protein deposits. (To help you remember, perform this procedure on the same day every week—the first or the last day, or every Wednesday, etc.) Once deposits are established, they will increase and can pit the lens surface, leaving it damaged even after it's purged of the accumulations. Enzyming is especially important for those who tend to produce tears heavily laden with protein. Factors such as air pollution, makeup, and eye irritation increase production of this protein.

The enzyme tablets come in a starter kit, which also contains two vials for mixing and soaking (one for each lens) and a "lens retriever" to help remove the lenses from the solution. After using up the starter tablets you can buy the tablets from your doctor or pharmacy and keep using the original vials and retriever.

To use the enzymatic cleaner follow the informative circular that the manufacturer provides with the package. Though the instructions suggest simply rinsing the lenses with saline before submerging the lenses in the enzyme solution, I would recommend that you use cleaning solution and rinse off the lenses thoroughly with saline. Also, instead of dissolving the enzyme tablet in distilled water, you may use premixed saline solution if you don't have distilled water on hand.

If you are allergic to the chemicals in preserved saline, I still recommend enzyming the lenses once a week and using the heat method of disinfection. If the chemicals in the enzyme cleaner affect your eyes, you can leach the lenses by soaking them in pure, unpreserved saline for several hours after enzyming.

LUBRICATING SOLUTIONS

Soft lenses are generally more comfortable than hard lenses. But an eye that's even slightly dry can cause soft-lens discomfort. To restore adequate moisture you can instill a drop or two of saline solution while wearing the lenses. Or you can use one of the special lubricating solutions formulated for contact lenses. These will clean, lubricate, and cushion the lenses while they're still in your eye, and may be used as often as needed. Decongestants, which are not formulated for contact lens use, contain chemicals that may be absorbed by the lenses and are definitely to be avoided. Never use any eye drops not recommended by your doctor while you are wearing soft contact lenses.

MECHANICAL CLEANING

Mechanical cleaning (massaging the lens with saline) is very important to maintain the integrity of the lens. If this procedure is omitted, a light filmy deposit will form on the lens, especially if it is heat disinfected. The lens will eventually become less comfortable, less transparent, and allow less oxygen to pass through it. In just a few weeks the lens will have to be replaced. Mechanical cleaning, therefore, is integral to every soft-lens wearer's regimen. For some wearers, however, it is the only method recommended for cleansing their lenses.

The surfactant cleaners, chemical disinfecting solutions, and preserved saline solutions all contain chemicals that the soft plastic lenses can absorb and then release into the eye. As previously stated, about 20 percent of soft-lens wearers are allergic to preservatives and therefore should not use the solutions that contain them. Usually switching to nonpreserved saline solution and thermal disinfection will solve the problem.

Such was the case with one of my patients. She had been using the cold disinfection method for a few months with no problems. One day she walked into my office with red, itchy, irritated eyes and a whitish ocular discharge. After purging her lenses of the chemicals, I placed her on a strict, no-preservative regimen that utilized a mechanical cleaning method, an unpreserved saline solution that she mixed herself, thermal sterilization, and once-a-week enzyming. Every day she removed her lenses, placed them one at a time in the palm of her hand, and placed several drops of the saline on the lens. She then massaged the lens with the index finger of her other hand for at least one minute to remove the accumulated dirt. After rinsing the lens with nonpreserved saline, it was ready for heat sterilization. This procedure has proved so successful, I now prescribe it for most of my allergic patients.

INSERTING SOFT CONTACT LENSES

There are various methods used to insert contact lenses. Your doctor will instruct you in the method he thinks is the easiest and most natural for you. Regardless of method, you will have to learn to overcome the natural tendency to blink as you insert the lens.

The first step in inserting a lens is to remove it from its case and rinse it with saline; this is especially important if you use chemical disinfecting solution. Place the lens on the tip of the finger, concave side up. Since the lens is so flexible, you may have easily flipped it inside out during cleaning and rinsing. Be careful to check the lens to make sure it's right side out. To do this you should place the lens, concave side up, on the tip of your finger. Check the profile; if the edges are straight up or turned in slightly, the lens is correct and ready for insertion. If it's inside out, the edges will flare out slightly. If you're still not sure, you can pinch the lens between thumb and forefinger. If the edges bend toward each other easily like a Mexican taco, the lens is correct. If it's not, the edges will flare out.

Place the lens on your saline-moistened fingertip, give it one last check to see that there are no foreign particles on the surface, and it's ready to insert using one of the following methods. (Reverse directions if you're left-handed.) After insertion blink firmly a few times to help the lens "settle." If there are any air bubbles under the lens, massage it gently

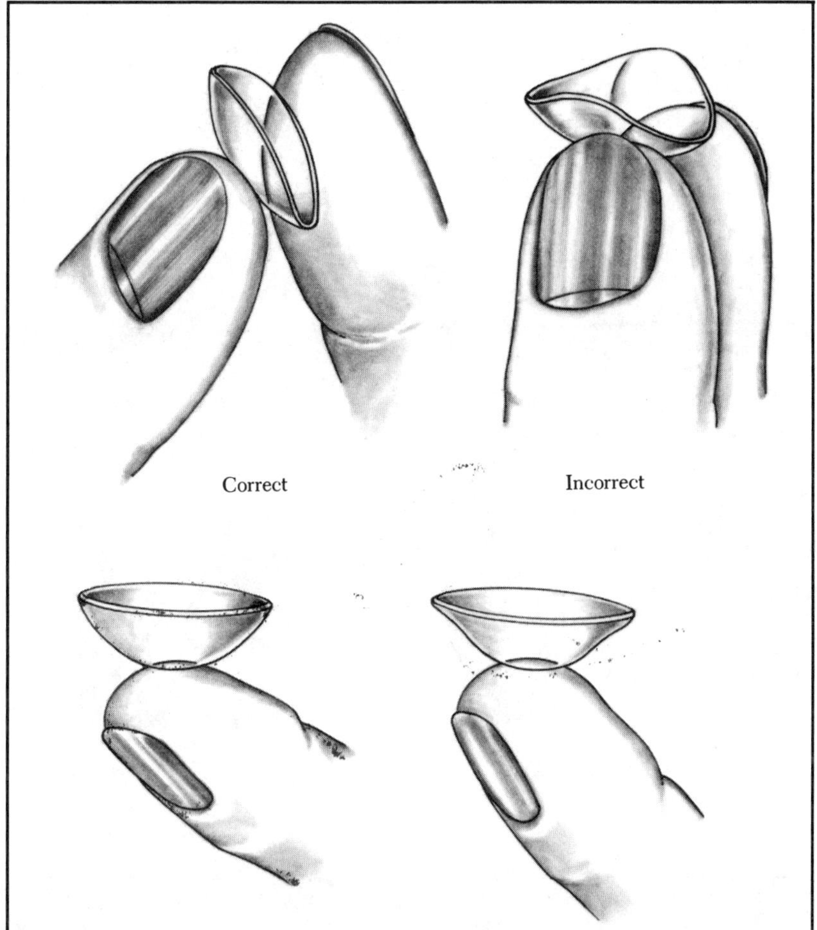

Figure 18. Checking the profile of a soft lens before insertion.

through the closed lids and blink hard a few times to remove the bubbles.

METHOD #1

1. Wet the tip of the index finger of the right hand with saline.

2. Place the lens, concave side up, on the tip of that finger.

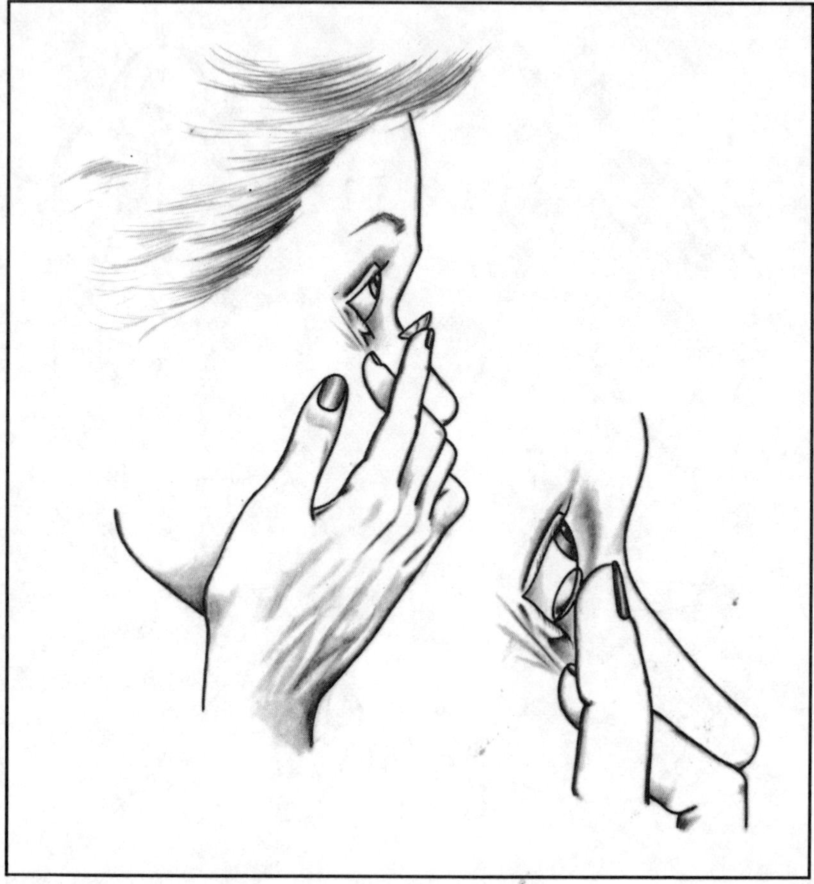

Figure 19. Inserting soft contact lens—Method #1.

3. With the middle finger of the right hand, pull down the lower lid.

4. Look up.

5. Place the lens on the white part of the eye, below the cornea. Make certain that the lens is on the eye and not adhering to your finger.

6. Release the lower lid and blink firmly.

7. Gently massage the lens with eyelids closed.

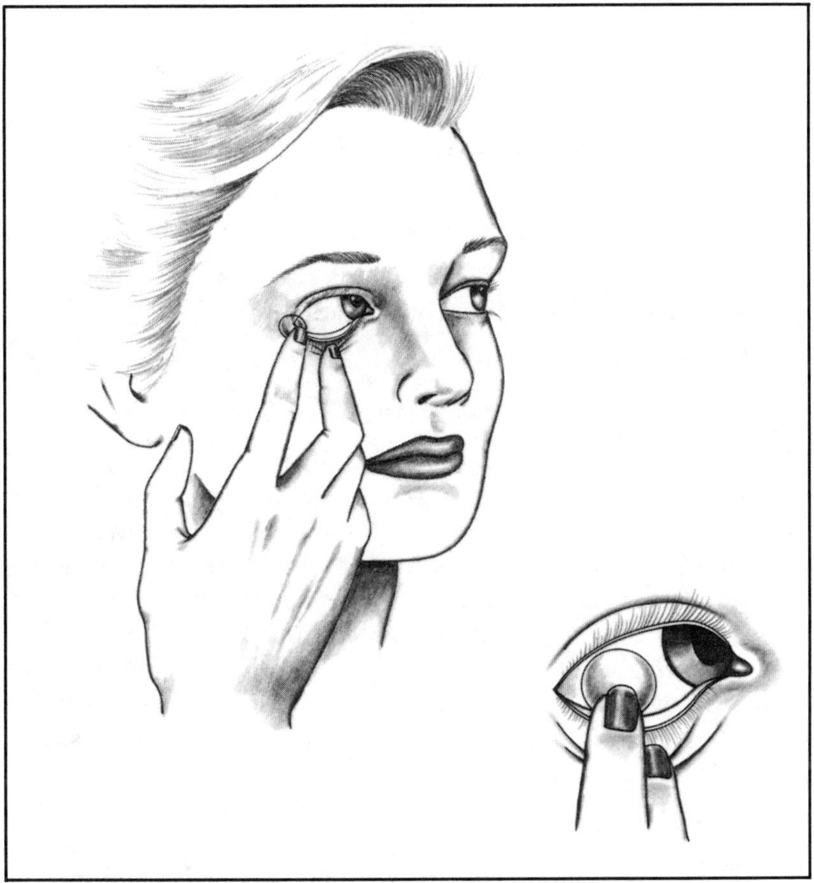

Figure 20. Inserting soft contact lens—Method #2.

METHOD #2

Same as Method #1 except that you:

1. Look toward your nose.

2. Place the lens on the white of the eye that is exposed (between the cornea and the outer part of the eye).

METHOD #3

1. Place the lens on the tip of the middle finger of the right hand.

2. Elevate the upper lid with the index finger of the right hand.

3. Retract the lower lid with the thumb of the right hand.

4. Place the lens directly on the cornea.

5. Release the eyelids.

CENTERING SOFT CONTACT LENSES

It's rare for a soft lens to decenter off the cornea because it clings so well to the surface of the eye. However, it can happen —usually when it is inserted or removed incorrectly. If you suspect a lens is off center, cover the other eye; if the vision is blurred, it means the lens isn't on the cornea. This is no cause for alarm; the lens cannot get lost behind the eye because of the anatomical barriers discussed previously. The lens will not harm the eye; theoretically it could remain on the sclera for days without adverse effects. However, a decentered lens does your vision no good.

METHOD #1

Close your eyelids and rotate your eyeballs in both directions. The lens should automatically recenter itself over the cornea.

METHOD #2

Close the eyelids and look down. Gently massage the lens onto the cornea through the closed upper eyelid, using the tip of your index finger.

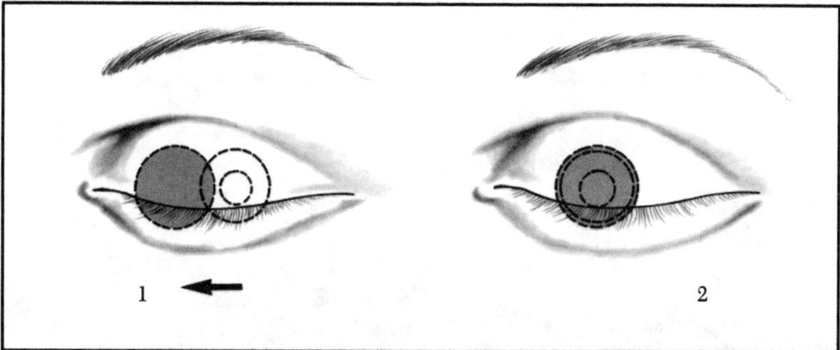

Figure 21. Centering soft contact lens—Method #1.

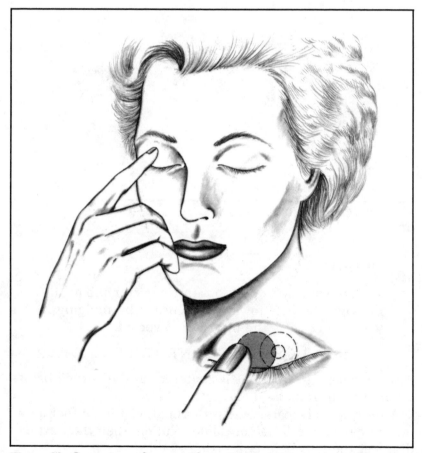

Figure 22. Centering soft contact lens—Method #2.

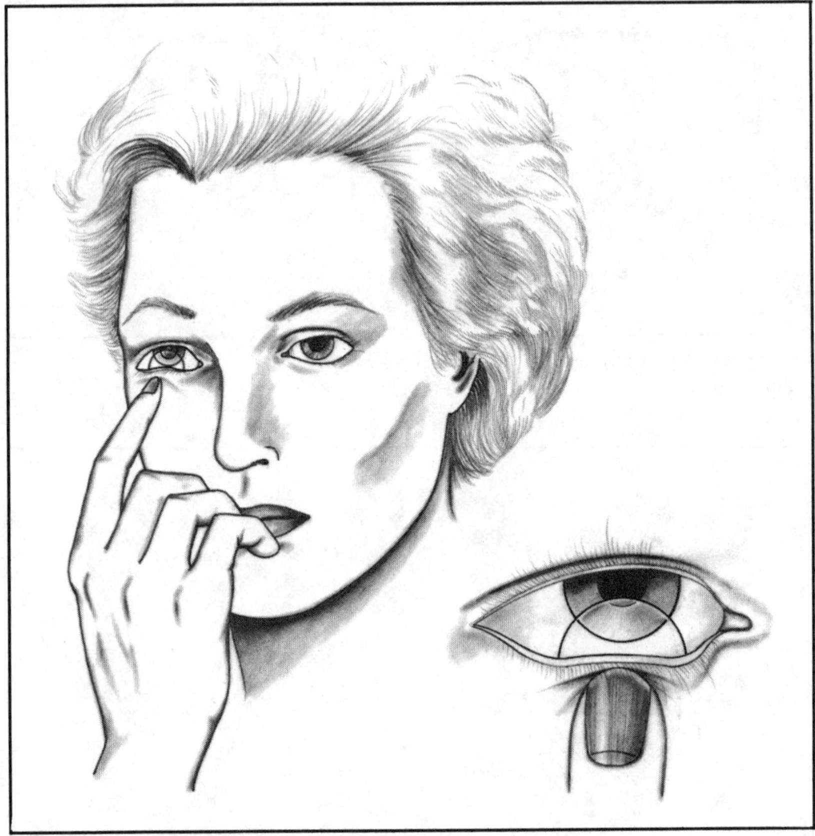

Figure 23. Centering soft contact lens—Method #3.

METHOD #3

With the eyes left open, look into a mirror and gently massage the lens toward the cornea by nudging it with the edge of the upper or lower lid.

REMOVING SOFT CONTACT LENSES

Always make sure the lens is centered on the cornea before attempting to remove it.

After removal clean the lens thoroughly, using either a surfactant cleaning solution or saline solution; then the next day disinfect the lens before inserting again.

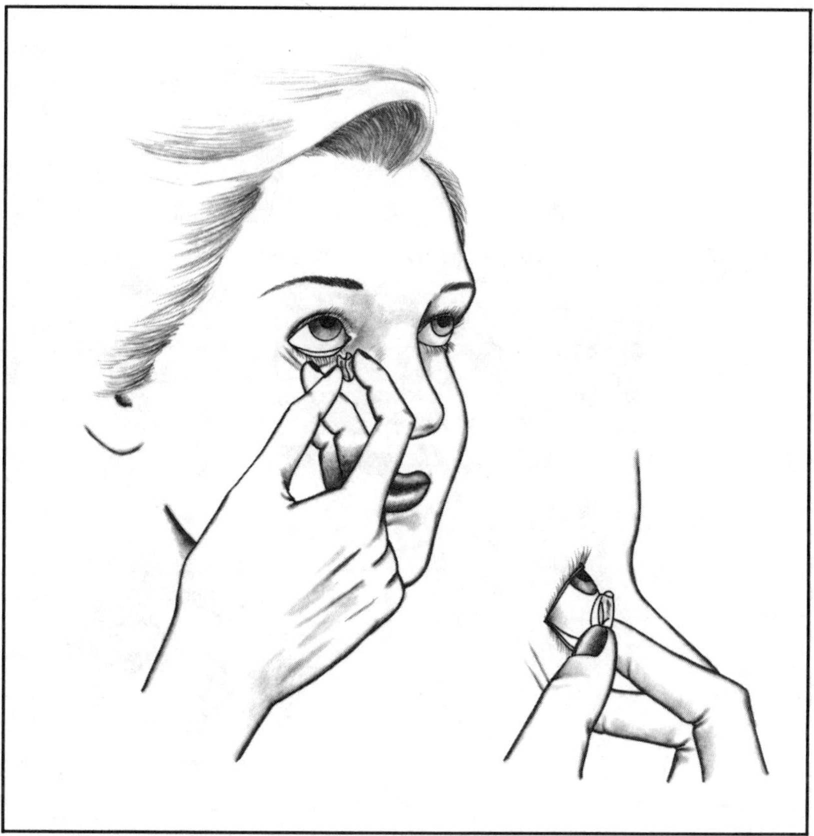

Figure 24. Removing soft contact lens—Method #1.

METHOD #1

1. Look up and open eyelids wide.

2. Pull the lower eyelid down with the middle finger of the right hand.

3. Place the tip of the index finger of the right hand on the lens.

4. Slide the lens down onto the white of the eye.

5. With the thumb and index finger of the right hand, gently fold or pinch the lens together.

6. Remove the lens.

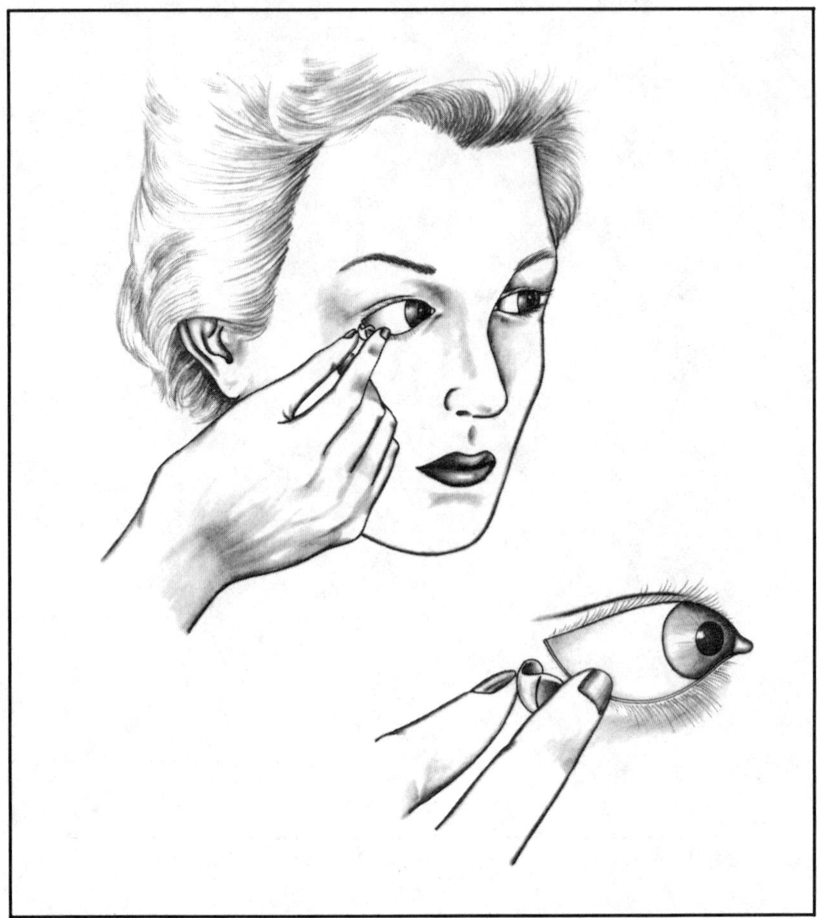

Figure 25. Removing soft contact lens—Method #2.

METHOD #2

Same as Method #1 except that you:

1. Look toward the nose.

2. Place the tip of the index finger of the right hand on the lens.

3. Slide the lens to the right of the eye toward the outer corner of the eye.

4. Pinch the lens together and remove it.

CHAPTER FIVE

GAS-PERMEABLE CONTACT LENSES

"Contact lenses and I are old friends: I started wearing hard contacts over fourteen years ago. I was amazed at the way they gave me instant beauty. Would you believe I never knew I had green eyes until I put on my first pair of contacts? But my life changed, and I began to get more and more annoyed with the discomfort; eventually I stopped wearing them. I thought: Why bother?

Then one day I decided it was time to be beautiful again. I'd heard about advances in the contact lens field, and concluded it was worth another try.

In spite of my determination I approached my eye doctor with a touch of trepidation. I'd gotten even more nearsighted over the years, and I half expected him to shake his head sadly and fit me with a cane and cup of pencils instead of contact lenses. We discussed soft lenses at first, but it turned out I have too much astigmatism for them. The alternative was gas-permeable contacts. I must admit they do feel more comfortable than my original lenses. They didn't feel as thick and bulky, and now it seems I'm bothered by fewer specks getting under them. Though I wear them almost every day, what I'm most grateful for is the fact that they give me the option to switch back to eyeglasses on the days I just don't want to bother with contacts."

Gas-permeable contact lenses are relatively new on the market, since 1979, and represent a major advance in the field.

They may eventually do for conventional hard contacts what soft lenses began to do more than a decade ago: that is, give them a good, hard shove toward extinction. But not only are hard lenses in danger of going the way of the dinosaur; soft lenses are getting a run for their money as well. The reason for this is that gas-permeable contacts offer many of the advantages of both hard and soft lenses, with few of their disadvantages. As an in-between kind of lens (one manufacturer even calls its lenses the Greek word *meso* for "in between"), it seems to offer the best of both worlds. And though no lens yet exists that is problem free, gas-permeable lenses fill the gap between conventional hard and soft lenses, and can often be worn successfully by those who aren't suited for any other type of lens.

Gas-permeable contact lenses are also known as oxygen permeable, semisoft, semihard, semirigid, or flexible lenses. As their names suggest, they are more flexible than conventional hard lenses, but less pliable than soft ones; and they are made from materials that allow oxygen and the waste gas carbon dioxide to pass through them. When the cornea can "breathe," it experiences no edema (swelling), which causes discomfort, and there is very little distortion of the vision after the lenses are removed (spectacle blur). The eye remains healthier, even when the lenses are worn for long periods of time. Contrast this with conventional hard (PMMA) lenses, which allow virtually no oxygen to pass through them, and with soft lenses, which allow some oxygen to pass through via the tears they absorb (but less oxygen than passes through gas-permeable material via the atmosphere).

Gas-permeable lenses offer the soft lens's main advantage: comfort and longer wear without sacrificing the health of the cornea; and the hard lens's main selling point: good visual acuity.

There are basically three types of gas-permeable lenses that are commercially available, with several brands still in the testing stage. They are either made of cellulose acetate butyrate (CAB), of silicone, or of silicone combined with PMMA, the same monomer used to make conventional hard lenses. Though they share the ability to transmit oxygen, the three materials have a host of differences:

CAB CONTACT LENSES
(Cellulose Acetate Butyrate)

These are the original gas-permeable lenses, and most of the brands of gas-permeable lenses on the market are made of CAB. CAB was developed in the 1930s by George Eastman for use in photography. It is an organic compound created from wood, cotton, vinegar, and natural gas; it is moderately stable, nontoxic, nonallergenic, optically clear, and fairly easily worked (though not as easily as silicone).

CAB lenses don't spring back into shape as readily as silicone lenses, so they tend to warp if they aren't handled carefully. When they are handled properly, though, they can last longer than lenses made with silicone. Even though they can be scratched, minor abrasions can be polished away. Although tests show that CAB, silicone, and PMMA/silicone are nearly equal in gas permeability, CAB is softer and less stable and requires that lenses be made thicker than PMMA/silicone lenses of equal prescription. The thicker the lens, the less gas passes through from the atmosphere. (Bear in mind that we are talking about fractions of millimeters.) On the other hand CAB is a highly wettable material (see p. 55), which increases the tear exchange and adds comfort. This increased tear flow may in fact contribute a great deal of oxygen to the cornea and is consequently a factor in the reduced amount of edema seen in eyes wearing CAB lenses. Furthermore this material reduces the temperature buildup beneath the lens; a cooler eye reduces the cornea's need for oxygen because the greater the heat buildup, the more oxygen is used.

SILICONE CONTACT LENSES

Silicone is not a plastic—it is a synthetic *rubber* that is flexible, stable, nontoxic, nonallergenic, has good optical quality, and is easily worked. The main attraction of the pure silicone lens, such as Dow Corning's Silsoft™ lens, which was the first 100 percent silicone lens to be FDA approved, is that it is completely oxygen permeable and the optics are excellent, providing sharp visual acuity. But there are drawbacks: It is very hydrophobic (does not absorb water); the lenses are quite thick and heavy, resulting in a sensation similar to that of hard

(PMMA) lenses; and protein and lipid deposits build up very rapidly on the lens surface and are very difficult to remove. To make the surface of a pure silicone lens wettable, it must be specially treated. Unfortunately, whenever any attempt to polish or modify the lens is made, the treated surface is removed. Though technically feasible, it is impractical to resurface such lenses, and they must be discarded.

SILICONE PLUS PMMA CONTACT LENSES

To utilize silicone for contact lenses some manufacturers combine it with PMMA. This hybrid material is being touted as the first substance ever developed specifically for contact lenses. When silicone is combined with PMMA, the desirable qualities of both materials are retained: wettability, durability, stability, and thinness from the PMMA and gas permeability from the silicone.

Since silicone/PMMA lenses don't have to be coated to make them more wettable, they can be modified and polished to remove minor surface scratches. This material is also quite pliable and bounces easily back into shape after flexing, which makes warpage less of a problem.

This lens can also be ground thinner (0.10 mm center thickness) than CAB because the material is more stable. Though both materials allow the same percentage of gas to be transmitted, the thinner design of silicone/PMMA lenses allows more oxygen to pass through them directly from the atmosphere. About one half the needed oxygen passes through the lens material itself; the other half is supplied by the tear-pump mechanism. The edges of this type of lens can also be kept thin, which adds to their comfort.

Unfortunately the surface tends to accumulate protein and other tear deposits, resulting in decreased permeability, comfort, and visual acuity. These deposits, though annoying, can usually be removed by the wearer. I advise using a tiny amount of 70 percent alcohol applied to the lens surface and gently rubbing the lens between the thumb and index finger to remove stubborn deposits. Afterward, use cleaning and soaking solutions as usual.

Many experts are looking hopefully toward the future developments in this exciting new type of contact lens. For instance, because of the high gas permeability, these lenses are being tested for extended wear and they may eventually compete for this market as well. At present, however, none have been FDA approved for this purpose, though one lens (the pure silicone) has been FDA approved for extended *aphakic* (following cataract extraction) wear. Of course the problem of protein deposits remains to be solved. More down-to-earth expectations include a larger variety of designs to fit more people, and increased permeability.

WHO SHOULD WEAR GAS-PERMEABLE CONTACT LENSES

This type of contact lens fills the need for many people who—for one reason or another—are not suitable for conventional hard or soft lenses. This is the lens for you if you:

- Have found hard lenses uncomfortable, but are unwilling to give up their sharp visual acuity.
- Would like a contact lens that approaches soft-lens comfort, but cannot wear soft lenses because of astigmatism or "dry eye."
- Like the idea of increased wearing time, but cannot wear soft lenses.
- Can't handle soft lenses.
- Can wear soft lenses but don't like the inconvenience involved in the care.
- Are interested in the possibilities of part-time lens wear, but can't wear soft lenses.

ADVANTAGES OF GAS-PERMEABLE CONTACT LENSES

These lenses offer a unique blend of the advantages of both hard and soft lenses. They provide excellent visual acuity, and correct most types of astigmatism better than soft lenses (but not quite as well as conventional hard lenses). The gas-permeable lenses correct astigmatism in the same manner as the hard lenses by forming a perfectly round, smooth inner surface filled with tears. Multifocal gas-permeable lenses are also available for the presbyope. They are almost as durable as hard lenses, and much more so than soft lenses. You can expect gas-permeable lenses to last up to five years. Since the lenses are firm in consistency, they are handled easily and with greater confidence than are soft lenses. They can be accurately reproduced, so there are none of the surprises that can occur when reordering a soft lens.

Because oxygen and carbon dioxide can pass directly through the material, the lenses can be worn in comfort for relatively long periods of time with no adverse effects on the cornea. Because the cornea can "breathe" better with these lenses than with conventional hard contact lenses, you have an easier break-in period. There is less chance of the overwear syndrome occurring; less corneal edema occurs (eliminated completely in some wearers); and the reduction in spectacle blur allows you to switch easily from contacts to glasses. There is less of the increased sensitivity to light which may occur with hard lenses.

Greater comfort and longer full-time wear are a boon to every hard-lens wearer but are especially important for those people with special visual defects such as *aphakia* or *keratoconus* (misshapen cornea), which can often be satisfactorily corrected only with hard lenses. Such people depend upon their contacts to a much greater extent than those who wear contact lenses for cosmetic purposes.

Because oxygen goes through the material itself, these lenses don't have to be as small as the hard lenses to enhance oxygen supply to the cornea. Though the size is a factor in the overall fit and comfort, gas-permeable lenses are often slightly larger in diameter than conventional hard lenses. This increase in lens surface gives you better night vision (when the pupil dilates) with none of the annoying—and possibly dangerous—halos or flare that plague the hard-lens wearer. Since the larger diameter makes the lens edge fit under the upper lid, there's less likelihood of the lens falling out.

You are also able to wear these lenses part time—only socially, or casually—the same as with soft lenses, thus saving them only for weekends, evenings, or other special occasions.

Irritation from foreign objects such as dust from the atmosphere is less of a problem with these lenses than with standard hard lenses. This is due to the thinness of the lens, which allows it to cling more tightly to the cornea and to the fact that the lens covers more of the cornea. Of course, at all times, the lens rides on a thin layer of tears.

DISADVANTAGES OF GAS-PERMEABLE CONTACT LENSES

Though the eventual comfort level is somewhere between that of a hard lens and a soft lens, a few wearers may complain of an initial scratchy sensation. Because of the nature of the materials, the lenses are often made slightly larger than conventional hard lenses. There are also difficulties in modifying and adjusting the fit of some of the lenses, and these lenses cannot be fenestrated successfully to relieve any dry-eye problem.

Astigmatism is not corrected quite as well as it is with conventional hard lenses. However, vision is appreciably sharper than with soft lenses, even the toric soft contacts.

Gas-permeable lenses are more expensive than hard lenses; they cost even more than conventional soft lenses. But since they are nearly as durable as hard lenses, replacement is less frequent. The lenses can, however, be chipped and scratched. Warping may occur with time, though damage is minimized with proper handling. CAB lenses can be stained by eye makeup and hairspray. The surface deposits that form easily on the silicone lenses can't always be removed completely with the usual cleaning and soaking solutions. This is less prevalent with the CAB lenses.

The lenses are difficult to make and delivery time may take a few weeks. The right lens cannot be dotted to avoid confusing the right and left lenses.

ADJUSTMENT AND WEARING TIPS

The eventual comfort of gas-permeable lenses lies somewhere between that of soft and hard lenses. Novice contact lens wearers will experience some of the initial foreign-body sensation similar to that of the hard lens, but the point at which they can be worn full time comes much sooner. In addition the number of hours meant by "full time" is longer: sixteen hours is common, as opposed to the eight that's usual for conventional hard

TYPICAL WEARING SCHEDULE—GAS-PERMEABLE CONTACT LENSES

Day 1

Two periods of two hours each with the lenses in place.

Day 2

Two periods of three hours each with the lenses in place.

Day 3

One period of five hours.

Day 4

One period of six hours.

Day 5

One period of seven hours.

Day 6

One period of eight hours.

Day 7

One period of nine hours.

lenses. Some who switch from conventional hard lenses to gas-permeable lenses are not initially impressed with the difference in comfort and wearing time, but this gradually improves as the eye recovers from the effects of wearing (and overwearing) their original hard lenses.

Continue adding one hour of wearing time each day until a maximum of sixteen hours is reached. If you wish to exceed the limit your practitioner has given you, make sure you get his permission.

In general, you can follow the wearing and adaptation tips suggested in Chapter Three, Hard Lenses. Even though these lenses permit more gas exchange than conventional hard lenses, by rights they should be called semi–gas permeable because, except for those made of pure silicone, they still don't allow 100 percent transmission of gases. Thus overwear can still occur, with its attendant edema, discomfort, and spectacle blur. Those for whom the lenses are exceptionally comfortable —even right away—are particularly in danger of being lulled into a false sense of security. In addition, the percentage of oxygen that reaches the cornea is lessened when the lenses become coated with mucus and deposits. Accumulation of protein deposits is one annoying habit that gas-permeable silicone lenses share with soft lenses. So is the tendency of CAB lenses to absorb undesirable substances such as cosmetics, hair sprays, and small amounts of the preservatives contained in the solutions used in their care.

CARE AND HANDLING OF GAS-PERMEABLE CONTACT LENSES

According to the present laws, the FDA classifies as a "drug" any contact lens that contains material other than the PMMA from which standard hard lenses are made. This includes, of course, all soft contact lenses; and since gas-permeable lenses contain either silicone or CAB, they fall into this category as well. The FDA feels that all the lenses in this class should be sterilized. Thus by FDA decree the manufacturers of gas-permeable lenses must recommend that you use the same regimen and solutions for cleaning, rinsing, and chemically disinfecting as with soft contact lenses. (Boiling, or heat disinfection, is not recommended, as the lenses would be ruined.) The literature that accompanies the lenses even warns, in large print, that unless you clean and disinfect the lenses daily, you may develop a "severe" ocular infection. However, I have not found this to be the case. In fact I have found that the solutions recommended by the FDA do not adequately clean the gas-permeable lenses and they may even produce some allergic reactions. Nor do they contain any wetting agents to make the lenses more comfortable on the eyes. And, as representatives from the gas-permeable lens manufacturers note, the hard-lens cleaners perform better in ridding some of the lenses of mucus buildup.

In reality gas-permeable lenses resemble hard lenses more than they do soft lenses. The materials from which they are made behave more like PMMA: they are hydrophobic (do not absorb water); they have a smooth, slick, small-pored surface that's more easily cleaned than soft lenses; and there's no reason to believe that infection is more of a danger than with hard lenses.

In the absence of solutions formulated specifically for gas-permeable materials many practitioners advise their patients to use hard-lens solutions for cleaning, wetting, and soaking their lenses, in spite of the fact that it has not been established to the FDA's satisfaction that these solutions are safe to use with these lenses. I recommend to my patients that they use Blairex Cleaner for cleaning, and Soaclens™ for soaking. Additionally, some wearers instill a few drops of a lubricating and cushioning solution before inserting the lenses; or they wet the lens with a few drops of Adapettes™ or Clerz™ lubricating solution. You should avoid solutions containing *chlorobutanol,* a preservative, if you have the silicone/PMMA type of gas-permeable lenses. This substance can bind to the silicone in the lens and cause discomfort.

Silicone/PMMA lens wearers may find that their lenses accumulate annoying protein deposits. Your practitioner will probably recommend that you treat your lenses to a once-a-week enzyming to remove these deposits. (See Soft Lenses, Chapter Four.) These deposits may also be removed by rubbing the lens surface with a little 70 percent rubbing alcohol, and then cleaning the lens as usual.

In addition mechanical cleaners such as Swirl Clean™ and Hydramat™ help in removing deposits that the fingertip can't reach, such as near the edges and at the very center.

INSERTION, REMOVAL, CENTERING

These techniques are the same for gas-permeable contact lenses as for conventional hard contact lenses (see Chapter Three).

CHAPTER SIX

EXTENDED-WEAR CONTACT LENSES

"I know it must sound crazy, but few things in life have ever looked so good to me as the pattern of paint cracks in my bedroom ceiling. That was the very first thing I saw when I opened my eyes the morning after I'd slept while wearing my new extended-wear contact lenses. Seeing those mundane little cracks meant that I really could wear the lenses overnight. It was a dream come true and, in a sense, my life hasn't been the same since.

Just before I got my new extended-wear lenses, the near-constant presence of big-city dirt and dust under my hard contact lenses had brought me to the verge of giving up lenses completely. I'd been wearing them for over ten years and was mighty tired of the old nightly and morning ritual too. At my next annual exam my doctor realized how unhappy I was and mentioned the availability of a new type of lens that was safe to wear while sleeping. He thought I'd be a good candidate; I nearly swooned with the good news . . . nearly fainted when I heard the price tag. But I decided to make the lenses a birthday present to myself.

That first night I slept with them in, I was so excited I had trouble falling asleep. When I did finally doze off, I kept waking up from anticipation. Part of it was fear too . . . I'd once napped while wearing hard lenses and didn't want to repeat the discomfort that followed that little accident. But these lenses can't compare. Though my eyes felt a little murky that first morning and still do sometimes, I just place a few drops of saline in them and everything clears up in few minutes. My vision isn't quite as sharp as it was with hard lenses, but I'll trade good consistent vision, convenience and comfort for 20/10 vision anytime. You're listening to someone who needed glasses at the age of nine, and for whom groping around an ill-lit unfamiliar room is practically a life-threatening experience. Now I take good, round-the-clock vision for granted. Other people find it hard to believe I wear contact lenses; I do, too. Only the once-a-week removal, cleaning, disinfecting, and re-insertion remain to remind me of what it's like to be unable to see well. Nothing is perfect, but these contact lenses come closest for me. It's like getting a new pair of eyes. I think they're worth every penny."

EXTENDED-WEAR SOFT CONTACT LENSES

Contact lenses that you can wear while you sleep—this earth-shattering concept arouses no less interest and excitement than the Pill did when it was first introduced. This is the glamour lens that everybody wants to know about and have, and is probably the lens of the future. Like the Pill, which forever altered our sexual standards, the extended-wear contact lens promises to usher in a new era and change our attitudes toward visual correction. But the similarity doesn't end there: Though this lens seems to be the answer to every contact lens wearer's prayers, it has not yet been perfected. It is definitely not for everyone, and some practitioners are reluctant to prescribe it at all.

Canada, Australia, and Europe enjoyed several types of extended-wear contact lenses several years before we did. However, there is no Food and Drug Administration in those parts of the world, and because of this lack of strict monitoring control and quality, these lenses have posed a health problem, especially as related to corneal complications.

In the United States the Food and Drug Administration, the watchdog for all non-PMMA contact lenses, places rigorous restrictions and guidelines on such lenses. At first the only type of extended-wear lenses that the FDA approved were therapeutic bandage lenses worn on the cornea and the sclera for use in treating certain eye disease (see Chapter Seven, Special Lenses). However, the potential of these lenses for correcting refractive errors was soon realized, and eventually the FDA allowed a few contact lens manufacturers to produce extended-wear corneal lenses. A handful of qualified ophthalmologists and optometrists were then permitted to fit and investigate the extended-wear lenses as visual corrective devices.

In 1978 they were approved for wear by aphakes (those people who have undergone cataract extraction; see Chapter Seven) since they have a pressing need for an alternative to the often unsatisfactory spectacles and available contact lenses. Then in 1980, after five years of rigorous testing by a select group of ophthalmologists (of which I was one) and optometrists on a specially selected group of volunteer patients, the first two brands of extended-wear contact lenses were approved for general cosmetic use: Perma-Lens, fabricated from perfilcon A, a terpolymer, and made by Cooper Vision; and Hydrocurve II, composed of the polymer bufilcon A, and made by Continuous Curve, Inc., and Revlon.

The reaction of the eye to extended contact lens wear is even more important than in daily-wear contact lenses. The lenses must allow plenty of oxygen to reach the cornea because the cornea does not have the same opportunity to recover from prolonged oxygen deprivation as it does with daily-wear contact lenses. In addition, during sleep the eyelids are closed so the ocular physiology is different: there is no available oxygen from the atmosphere and there is an absence of oxygen-filled tears. The semirigid gas-permeable lenses (see Chapter Five) would logically seem to fit the bill for optimum oxygen supply, but studies so far have revealed drawbacks in these lenses during prolonged wear. Except for the pure silicone lenses used by aphakes, the contact lenses that have been FDA approved to date for extended wear are all soft, and made of plastics similar to those from which conventional soft lenses are made, but modified to yield greater oxygen permeability. The rate of oxygen–carbon dioxide transmission through the lens material is determined by two major factors: the water content and the thickness of the lens. The higher the percentage of water contained in the lens material, and the thinner the lens, the more gas is exchanged. A very thin, very high-water-content lens, however, has so far proven to be too fragile to be practical. Thus, a lens manufacturer can take either of two roads to maximize gas transmissibility. It can design a relatively thick lens with a high water content (Perma Lens), or a very thin lens with a lower water content (Hydrocurve II).

Extended-wear lenses are therefore from 55 percent (Hydrocurve) to 75 percent (Perma-Lens) water. Conventional daily-wear soft lenses are on the average about 30 to 40 percent water. The Hydrocurve extended-wear contact lens is as thin as a single strand of hair (0.05 mm).

Oxygen transmissibility is not the only factor in lens wear, however, and thickness and water content not the only variables. The different materials have different properties, and there are different diameters, edge designs, and other design factors to be considered. For instance, the lower the water content of a lens, the higher the tensile strength it has, and the less it tends to accumulate deposits and support the growth of bacteria and fungus. This can mean a longer useful lens life, more comfort, and less frequent replacements. Lower water content yields a slightly more rigid lens, which generally provides better visual acuity. On the other hand the higher the water content, the softer will be the lens and the more comfortable it may feel. But the higher the water content, the more important it is to have adequate tear flow, since the tear flow is essential to keep the lens hydrated. Thinner lenses are more apt to fold and tear and are more difficult to handle. Also, it may be difficult to determine whether they have inverted or not.

Even with more than one brand to choose from, it is impossible to predict whether someone will be able to wear contact lenses for an extended period of time. The cornea and tear composition of each person are different, as is the tendency to form protein deposits and the ability of the eye to adapt to life with less oxygen and a diminished tear pump. It is up to the doctor to weigh the obvious benefits against the possible risks to the health of the eye. Now that extended wear has been FDA approved, any eye practitioner can dispense them, regardless of how much (or how little) experience he has had with them. This is the most promotable form of contact lens wear by far, and the media exposure can sometimes paint too pretty a picture, giving the consumer unrealistic expectations. It is especially important to have a highly experienced ophthalmologist monitor the health of your cornea during extended contact lens wear. True success comes only with strict supervision. Patients must understand the importance of compliance with a strict follow-up schedule of numerous eye examinations, during which subtle changes in the eye may be discovered, indicating that extended wear must be stopped.

Any sign of a problem (red eyes, reduced vision, discharge, or irritation) should be reported to the doctor at once and the lenses should be removed immediately. Reinsertion of the lenses should occur only after your doctor has made certain that your eyes have returned to their normal, healthy state.

ADVANTAGES OF EXTENDED-WEAR CONTACT LENSES

Because they are so thin and have such a high water content, extended-wear contacts are even more comfortable than daily-wear soft lenses. Since they are worn round the clock, your vision is corrected all day, from the minute you awaken until the minute you close your eyes. You're able to read the alarm clock whenever you need to with no more groping for eyeglasses, and you can fall asleep while watching TV or while reading a book. You can even swim with these lenses, providing you don't dive into the water or keep your eyes wide open. However, as mentioned in the chapter on soft lenses, you should remove them if you plan to swim in a chlorinated pool. Travelers especially appreciate the convenience of not having to remove and clean their lenses nightly. There is no extra bulk and weight of contact lens accessories to lug around during trips. They are a particular boon to campers, who often have to abandon their soft lenses while roughing it.

Patients who have difficulty or are nervous about insertion, removal, cleaning, and handling contact lenses enjoy a tremendous reduction in these problems. This is of special importance for the person who has undergone cataract extraction, or who has a physical disability such as arthritis or tremors. But it's also a tremendous time-saver for those with busy schedules or who just don't want to bother with the daily routine of caring for contact lenses. An important aspect is the fact that there's less risk of tearing the lens since handling of the lenses is reduced. There is also less chance of an allergic reaction to preservatives in the solutions since the lenses and the eyes are exposed to them less often. Finally the initial costs are somewhat offset by the less frequent use of contact lens solutions and the lower incidence of lost or damaged lenses.

DISADVANTAGES OF EXTENDED-WEAR CONTACT LENSES

Compared with conventional soft lenses, the extended-wear lenses offer almost all the same liabilities , as well as a few more. They are the most expensive contact lenses (about six hundred dollars), in part because of the cost of the special lenses but mainly because of the extensive professional follow-up examinations required.

The visual acuity provided by the extended-wear lenses is similar to that of conventional daily-wear soft lenses. So far these lenses are available only for those who are nearsighted and for those who have undergone cataract extraction. They cannot correct significant amounts of astigmatism. However, research is going on in this field.

Extended-wear contacts will absorb impurities from the environment and are even more prone than conventional soft lenses to accumulate deposits of lipid, protein, calcium, and mucus from the tears and eyelids. In some cases these deposits simply cannot be removed, and the lenses must be replaced.

Extended-wear lenses are less durable than other lenses and may have to be replaced as often as twice a year. Though they are inserted and removed infrequently, a delicate touch is required. Many people have difficulty in handling the lenses since the extended-wear lenses have the feel and consistency of Saran Wrap. It is also extremely difficult to tell whether these lenses are inside out. Usually the best candidates for extended-wear lenses are those who have previously worn lenses—particularly soft lenses—on a daily basis. These wearers are familiar with the normal sensations that conventional soft lenses produce and are thus in a better position to detect and report abnormal symptoms to their eye doctor. In fact, when I fit an individual with extended-wear lenses, I make certain that he has gone through at least one week of daily insertion and removal.

Though for the most part wearers can forget about their lenses while they're wearing them, extended-wear lenses may become uncomfortable under certain conditions. Dry air can do it; so can the accumulation of the aforementioned deposits. A reduction in oxygen supply can result from extended wear, producing irritation and edema, since some eyes simply need more oxygen than others—especially when the contact lens is worn for long periods of time.

In some cases round-the-clock contact lens wear may temporarily thicken and distort the cornea, resulting in spectacle blur whenever the contacts are removed and glasses are worn. In rare instances extended wear may increase the chance of infection. In the first place wearers are sometimes lulled into a false sense of security because the lenses stay on for so long. They may forget that they are, in fact, contact lens wearers, and become cavalier in their attitude toward caring for their lenses and their eyes. If an infection should occur, it happens under the lens "bandage" and may not be as evident as in daily-wear lenses. Reduced tear flow and oxygen supply may cause the surface of the cornea to become swollen and even abraded, providing a welcome mat for microbes and bacteria that will multiply even more readily when there's less air in their environment. On the other hand, in daily wear a slight infection that's taken hold can be halted at an early stage when the lens is removed, the cornea is exposed to the air, and the normal supply of bacteria-fighting tears is present.

Since 1975, when I was chosen to be a research investigator for one of the extended-wear contact lens companies, I have had the opportunity to fit many patients with these lenses. Despite rigid written and oral instructions as to the care and handling of the lenses, the need for frequent eye examinations, and the attention to abnormal symptoms, there was a small percentage of patients with poor compliance—and therefore poor lens performance. Such was the case of one patient who, even after suffering for several days, thought that a red, irritated eye was not important enough to bring to my attention. When she did finally arrive at my office, she had a severe corneal ulcer. The lens was immediately removed and she was placed on antibiotic drops and oral medication. The healing process took two weeks, and she was fortunate that the infection cleared fully, leaving no permanent scar.

Keratitis, characterized by tiny areas of abrasion or inflammation on the surface of the cornea, can occur in any type of contact lens wear, but is more common in extended wear. A decrease in oxygen supply may be the cause, or the cornea may become irritated by the contact lens solutions used, or by the lens itself when the tear layer is too thin. The condition may also be the result of infection.

Another potential hazard with extended wear is *neovascularization,* a growth of new blood vessels on the normally *avascular* (without blood vessels) cornea. This results because a reduction in oxygen stimulates the formation of new blood vessels as the body attempts to restore the supply of this vital gas. By reducing the oxygen supply sufficiently over a significant period of time, extended-wear contact lenses are the lens type most likely to create this condition. Neovascularization will cause eye irritation and reduce visual acuity. However, the blood vessels will disappear after the lenses have been removed.

Wearers must bear in mind that these are *extended wear* (days, weeks, months) contact lenses, not *continuous wear.* Though they have been approved by the FDA for up to two weeks for cosmetic wear, and three months or more for aphakes, the schedule will vary from person to person. How long you go between cleanings depends upon the health of your eyes, the amount of lens deposits you tend to accumulate, the type of lens, the way you work and relax, your individual ocular physiology and tear chemistry, and even the environment in which you live and work. (City air is not a particular problem, but confined areas of fumes, gases, and sprays are a contraindication for wearing any type of contact lens.) Naturally, specific instructions will be given to you by your doctor. In some patients the lenses simply become too dirty too rapidly to make extended wear feasible.

ADAPTATION AND WEARING TIPS

In general extended-wear patients follow similar instructions concerning adaptation and wear as outlined in the chapter on conventional soft contact lenses. The slight discomfort some experience at first usually disappears in a very short time; vision may fluctuate until the eye adjusts and the lens "settles in."

Other than that there's almost no adaptation time to speak of. Patients usually go on an extended-wear regimen after one week of daily wear.

Minor symptoms to be on the lookout for are excessive tearing, redness, stinging, burning, itching, blurry vision, halos around lights, and light sensitivity. If any of these occur, remove the lens for at least three hours. If the problem ceases, your lens may be the source of the problem and you should check to see if cracks or chipped or ripped edges are present. Do not reinsert the lens if it is damaged. Put it back in its case and return it to the doctor, who will order a replacement. If you see dirt or an eyelash (or any other foreign matter) use the enzyme solution, clean, and disinfect the lens. Then you may reinsert it. If any of these problems persist, consult your doctor.

FOLLOW-UP EXAMS

It's very important that you return to your eye practitioner for follow-up eye examinations. It is recommended that these occur:

- After the first twenty-four hours of extended wear.
- After the first three days of extended wear.
- After the first week of extended wear.
- After each month of the first six months of extended wear.
- After each six months of extended wear.

CARE AND HANDLING OF EXTENDED-WEAR CONTACT LENSES

The procedures used in extended-wear lens care and handling

are essentially the same as for conventional soft contact lenses. Instructions on inserting, removing, centering, cleaning, and disinfecting the lenses will be found in Chapter Four. The main modification is the frequency with which these are done. There are also a few additional amendments of which the extended-lens wearer should be aware that will make these lenses more comfortable and safer.

Lens deposits are the most frequent cause for discomfort and replacement. That these lenses are worn longer and are very high in water content encourages deposits to form even more readily than on conventional soft contact lenses. Proper care and hygiene are therefore even more important, and the diligent cleansing of extended-wear lenses adds appreciably to their useful life.

For cosmetic wear the lenses may be worn up to fourteen days. On the fourteenth night the lenses should be removed, cleaned with a surfactant and/or saline and enzyme solution, disinfected, and then reinserted the next morning. However, some patients find they must remove and clean their lenses more frequently. The patient can perform these procedures himself, except when he goes for checkup exams. At that time the lenses are removed, cleaned, and reinserted in the office by the doctor or his technicians.

Aphakes wear their lenses longer in general: from one month up to six months, with an average of three months of extended wear. These patients usually leave the cleaning procedures to the doctor, who performs them whenever the patient goes for a checkup. Sometimes a neighbor or relative can be instructed to clean, remove, and insert the lenses for the patient between office visits if the wearer is unable to do this for himself.

Extended-wear lenses may be disinfected either thermally or chemically. If the heat method is employed, a "low-heat" unit should be used to avoid shortening the life of the lenses.

LUBRICATING THE LENSES WHILE IN PLACE

Whenever the lenses feel dry, scratchy, or don't move freely on the eyes, relief may be obtained by instilling a few drops of saline solution or lubricating solution formulated for use with soft lenses. These eye drops may be used as often as you like.

They are especially helpful in the morning upon awakening when the eye and lens are their driest, and as a way to lubricate the lens before removal, since even a partially dehydrated lens can tear when it is removed.

For some, more involved measures are indicated in order to increase the comfort, slow down the progress of deposits, and reduce the incidence of "red eye." In between scheduled removals and cleanings you can give your eyes a saline bath while the lenses are in place. Dr. H. Johnson Kersley, the London ophthalmologist who devised this method, recommends that you use the unpreserved premixed saline solution, which comes in single-unit packets. Use one quarter of the packet in an eyecup for each eye, each morning and each night. (Thus one entire packet is used each day.) Apply the eyewash in the eyecup, keeping the lids partially closed, so that the eye, lids, and lashes are rinsed.

Alternatively, you could shower the eye and the lens by carefully and gently pouring a stream of saline into the open eye, head tossed back, blotting up the excess with a clean tissue.

These measures may help extend the length of time that the lenses can be worn without removal for cleaning. Even so, many extended-wear patients will have to remove and clean their lenses more often than every two weeks. A large number are on a once-a-week schedule, but even those who need to remove them every other day or every three days welcome the freedom from the inconvenience of daily care and the opportunity to lead fuller, more normal lives.

CHAPTER SEVEN

SPECIAL LENSES

BIFOCAL AND OTHER CONTACT LENSES FOR PRESBYOPIA

Eventually everyone experiences presbyopia. As explained in Chapter One, this is the normal aging process of the eye, which begins around the age of forty for most people, and is caused by the gradual loss of elasticity in the natural crystalline lens of the eye. The lens loses its ability to change shape the way it used to, and fails to bring the light rays of near objects into sharp focus. Of course a nearsighted person over the age of forty can see near objects clearly with the naked eye, but will have difficulty doing so if he is wearing glasses or contact lenses that correct his myopia.

The presbyope has "trombone vision"—that telltale gesture of moving objects farther and farther away from the eyes in order to see them clearly. Most people opt for bifocal glasses or simply resign themselves to placing on a separate pair of glasses to read, sew, and do other tasks that require good close-up vision. However, there are several ways to correct this condition with contact lenses: bifocal contact lenses, "monovision" lenses, "compromise" contact lenses, having two pairs of contact lenses, and wearing reading glasses over contact lenses.

BIFOCAL CONTACT LENSES

Currently in the U.S. bifocal contact lenses are available in two types: conventional hard lenses and the newly released soft lenses. There are available basically two designs of either form of bifocal contact lens. Both of these, like spectacles, have two distinct powers, or prescriptions: one for near, one for far.

Crescent bifocal contact lenses most resemble bifocal eye-

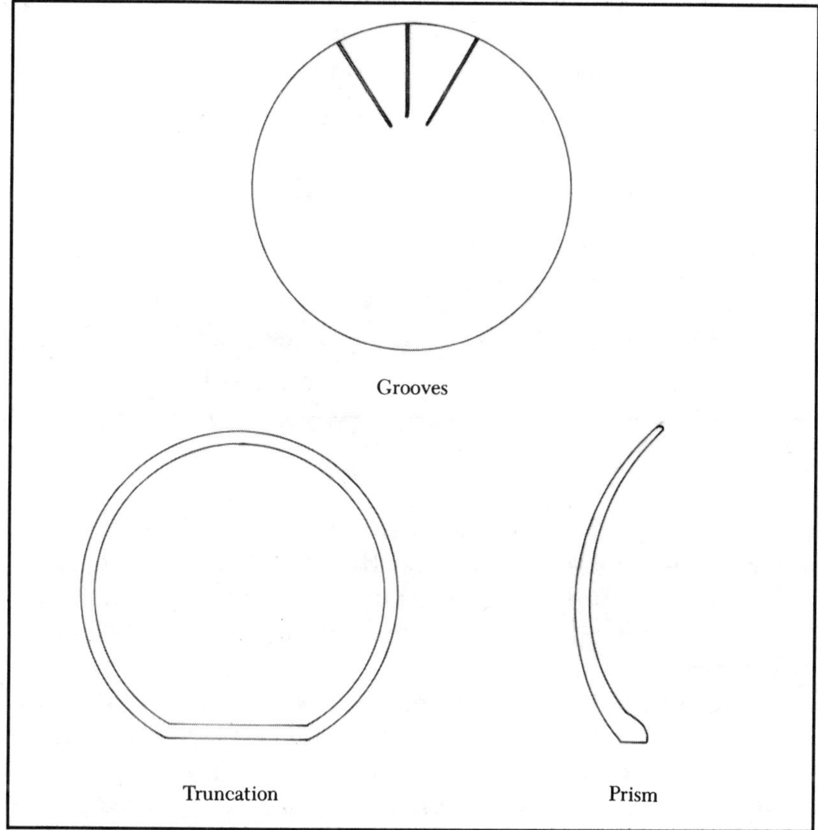

Figure 26. Methods of stabilization.

glasses. They have the prescription for distance at the top part of the lens, and the crescent-shaped segment at the bottom contains the prescription for close-up vision. As you gaze ahead normally, the distance power is used; as you gaze down, the near power goes into effect.

Because contact lenses naturally rotate on the eye during wear, some means of keeping bifocal lenses stabilized is necessary. Otherwise the crescent at the bottom would gradually drift toward the top where it would do no good—unless you held your newspaper over your head. These lenses are often weighted at the bottom with a thicker segment (*prism*), which utilizes gravity to keep the lens oriented. Crescent bifocals may also be *truncated*, a process in which the bottom edge is

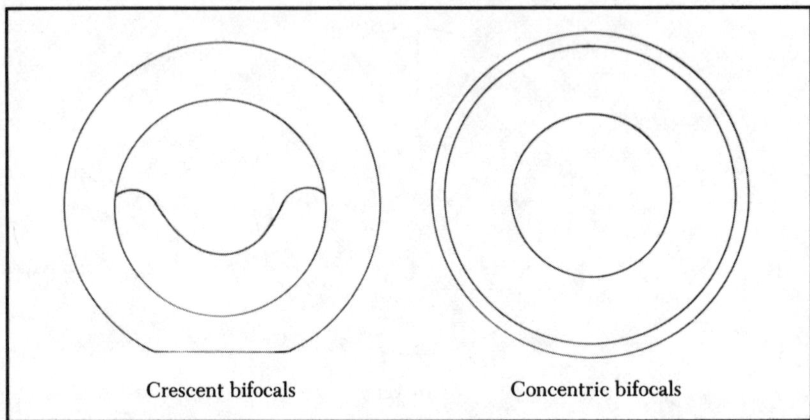

Figure 27. Types of bifocal contact lenses.

cut off to align it parallel with the lower eyelid margin. Another less effective modification that stabilizes bifocal lenses features *orientation grooves* cut into the top edge of the lens, providing a pathway for the inner surface of the upper lid to prevent rotation of the lens.

Like crescent lenses, *concentric bifocal contact lenses* also have two distinct powers, or prescriptions, but with a structural difference: the near prescription segment is in the shape of a ring acting as the outer rim of the lens; the distance power is a circle in the middle. With this lens, which resembles a bull's-eye target, there's no worry about its rotating on the eye. As with crescent bifocal lenses distant vision is effected by looking through the center, and near vision by looking down through the outer rim.

The best candidates for bifocal contact lenses are those who have been successfully wearing single-vision contacts for some time to correct myopia, hyperopia, or astigmatism. They will have the least problem with adjusting; but even so the success rate is low. The recent advent of the soft bifocal lens, however, should improve these statistics for the millions of presbyopes in this country, many of whom would no doubt be delighted to be able to wear bifocal contacts.

Fitting bifocal contact lenses is difficult (such factors as pupil size and lower lid position complicate the fitting process); manufacture of the lenses is more intricate than for the single-vision contacts; delivery time is slow; and the cost is necessarily higher than for conventional lenses. Many wearers report that bifocals are less comfortable than single-vision contacts, usually because the prism that prevents rotation adds bulk and makes the lens heavier. New contact lens wearers not only have to adjust to lens wear in general but also have to adjust to the means of wearing a bifocal prescription. As in bifocal spectacles this involves learning how to adjust to the "jump" in vision that occurs every time you shift your gaze from near to far, or vice versa. Initially vision may be frustratingly poor —especially with hard lenses—during the adaptation period because the sensation of having a foreign body in the eye causes ocular physiological changes that lift the lower lid and the lens. Thus the bifocal segment is higher than it should be. Since this bifocal segment is so very small, there is very little tolerance in the proper positioning of the lens. As difficult as it is to achieve, perfect centering of the contact lenses is absolutely crucial for successful bifocal hard contact lens wear.

In response to these problems manufacturers are experimenting with design modifications. *Multifocal* or *variable-focus* contacts (available in hard and gas-permeable lenses) have not two, but many powers that gradually blend into each other, avoiding the annoying jump in vision. The lens contains all the different powers needed by the wearer to see clearly at any distance: near, far, and intermediate. The bifocal contact lens candidate will have to be patient and well motivated because it usually takes a few weeks until the lenses can be worn with comfort and provide good vision. Also some lens modifications and adjustments are usually the rule.

MONOVISION CONTACT LENSES

In spite of these innovations bifocal contact lenses and their variations are obviously far from perfected. For those who can't be fitted, or who fail to adjust to bifocal lenses, there are a few alternatives and compromises. A very popular one and one that is extensively employed is the *"monovision* technique." One eye is fitted for distance (usually the dominant eye); the other is fitted for reading. Either hard or soft contact lenses may be used, and this is by far the best technique found to date: The success rate is estimated at between 70 and 80 percent. As in the past, when monocles were worn, the eyes and brain somehow manage to make sense out of what seems to be visual schizophrenia. Visual fusion and depth perception can still be obtained, and after a while the wearer forgets which eye has been corrected for distance and which for near. Though depth perception is usually adequate for normal wear, it is advised that a lens for distance be substituted for the reading lens during activities where depth perception is particularly important, such as driving or sports. With the monovision technique I have fitted many patients who are ecstatic about the fact that no glasses at all need to be worn.

COMPROMISE CONTACT LENSES

This method has two variations. One is to change the contact lens prescription for farsighted people so that both lenses are slightly stronger than needed for distance vision and slightly weaker than would be required for reading. Thus adequate—but not perfect—vision can be obtained at all distances. The second method is to undercorrect the contact lens prescription for the nearsighted person so that both lenses are slightly weaker than necessary for distance and slightly weaker than needed for reading. Again adequate, but not perfectly sharp, vision is obtainable for those patients who are ready to accept this compromise.

As with thc monovision technique the compromise technique may result in a small percentage of eyestrain or headaches. No permanent ocular damage can result; however, if the symptoms persist, this method should be discontinued.

TWO PAIRS OF CONTACT LENSES

This approach is useful for public speakers and others who require the ability to see close up while in the limelight. Having two pairs of contact lenses—one pair for distance vision and one pair for near—works well if you have the time and patience to switch from one set of lenses to the other.

GLASSES PLUS CONTACT LENSES

Of course there is always the option, whenever necessary, of wearing reading glasses for near vision over the distance-correcting contacts. This is still an improvement over wearing glasses for both refractive problems.

SOFT TORIC CONTACT LENSES TO CORRECT ASTIGMATISM

Conventional soft contact lenses cannot be used to correct moderate to large amounts of astigmatism. Their pliable nature causes them to conform to irregularities in the shape of the cornea and thus duplicate the astigmatic refractive error. Hard contact lenses are firm and hold their shape; they are able to correct high amounts of astigmatism because the spherical undersurface of the lenses and the tears beneath them create a new, smooth optical surface. Until recently, therefore, patients had two contact lens options: to either wear a hard lens and get sharp vision, or wear a conventional soft lens and live with less-than-perfect vision. Now there is a new type of soft contact lens, the toric lens, which give astigmatics a third choice. While it is still in the early stages of use and development, this lens will eventually be perfected, and will certainly be a part of the professional contact lens practitioner's armamentarium.

Currently the cost of such lenses is about half again as much as conventional soft lenses; they are technically difficult to manufacture; production and delivery tend to be slower than for conventional lenses; duplication is difficult; and they are trickier to fit. In addition, they don't always produce a favorable or predictable visual correction. This is due in part to the problem of lens rotation, which the toric lens shares with the bifocal lenses discussed earlier. As soon as the lens rotates on the eye, the axis of astigmatism becomes displaced and the vision becomes blurred, particularly when the astigmatism is severe. To solve this problem, a variety of solutions have been devised, similar to those used to stabilize bifocal contact lenses.

Most commonly, prisms are placed in the lower parts of the lenses; the added plastic orients the lens by using gravity to keep the lens in alignment. Or a small segment may be cut off the bottom of the lens; this truncation results in a straight edge that stays aligned and parallel with the edge of the bottom eyelid. A lens may have the top or bottom portions or both portions made especially thin so they remain aligned underneath the eyelids; this is known as slab off. Finally, orientation grooves, a series of tiny vertical lines, may be cut into the top edge of the lens. The inner surface of the upper eyelid crosses the grooves, and with each blink the lid pulls the lens toward the top, keeping the lens oriented.

CONTACT LENSES AFTER CATARACT SURGERY

Most people think that cataracts develop only in their grandparents. In fact, though the average patient is seventy years old, cataracts can occur in anyone from the time of birth to over one hundred years of age. Another misconception is that a cataract is a film growing over the eye, when in reality it is the natural, transparent, crystalline lens of the eye that becomes cloudy. The light rays passing through the cloudy lens become obstructed and vision becomes more and more blurred as the condition worsens. Most often cataracts are part of the normal aging process, but they may also be caused by injury, disease, birth defects, infection, vitamin deficiency, radiation, and enzyme deficiencies.

CATARACT SURGERY

The first step in restoring vision is to remove the cloudy lens surgically. This is one of the safest, most successful, and widely performed operations. Of the 400,000 to 600,000 cases performed annually in this country, over 90 percent succeed in helping to restore vision, thanks to improvements in surgical techniques and in the skills of ophthalmic surgeons.

The surgeon has a choice of several surgical approaches; the decision is based upon the type and stage of the cataract, as well as the age of the patient. The lens may be extracted by freezing the lens with a tiny metal probe that adheres to the cataract and removes it intact (cryoextraction). A relatively new method, ultrasonic phacoemulsification, employs a tiny titanium needle vibrating at forty thousand times per second that emulsifies the cataract, which is then aspirated through the same needle. The cataract incision may require several tiny sutures (in the cryoextraction technique) or only a single suture in the ultrasonic technique. The resulting postoperative condition of an eye without a lens is called aphakia; a person with aphakia is called an aphake. Aphakes are not blind as a result of surgery, but, because the normal refracting lens is gone, their vision is impaired (similar to what a normal person sees under water).

CATARACT EYEGLASSES

The next step in restoring sight is to provide a refracting lens to replace the normal crystalline lens which has been surgically removed. The traditional solution has been cataract eyeglasses. But these are heavy, and have thick "sunny-side-up" or "oyster" lenses that enlarge the visual image by 30 percent. Through these glasses the world looks strange and distorted. Peripheral vision is severely limited; the sensation is one of looking through a tunnel. Wearers often find that at first they spill things, or have trouble keeping their balance. Objects, such as doors, curve precipitously away or loom suddenly into view. The problem is compounded when only one eye has been operated on, and the patient has *monocular aphakia.* In this case only one eye receives the cataract eyeglass. It is almost impossible to correct monocular aphakia satisfactorily with glasses because the eyes can't work together: the images are of vastly different sizes, resulting in a lack of fusion or binocularity. This problem lasts until the other cataract is removed and that eye receives its own corrective spectacle. Consequently this solution is very rare these days. The main advantage of cataract glasses is the ease with which they can be put on and removed, and that they are a familiar, unthreatening device.

CONTACT LENSES

Contact lenses are, in most cases, a far better solution once the aphake is convinced that the "newfangled" device is worth trying. Advantages are the normal appearance of the eye and crisp visual acuity. Since only 6 percent magnification of objects occurs, the images appear to be of normal size, fusion can take place, and excellent peripheral vision and depth perception will result. Therefore life can go back to normal, the cosmetic effect is far better, and most observers can't tell that there's ever been a cataract extraction.

Daily-Wear Contact Lenses. Conventional hard lenses, gas-permeable lenses, and soft lenses can be worn to correct vision following a cataract removal. But the problem of daily insertion, removal, and cleaning is a real one, and discourages many a potential daily wearer. Fear of inserting a foreign object into the eye; diminished dexterity; reluctance to handle tiny, delicate, almost invisible objects—all can add up to a less-than-successful scenario. The replacement rate with soft lenses is particularly high: the average life span of a pair is two years because of loss, torn lenses, or lens deposits. Because of their advanced age aphakes often have dry eyes, and soft lenses require a more lavish tear supply than do hard lenses. Also, loose lids, usually found as a product of aging eye, can cause fitting and wearing problems.

Many aphakes do, however, adjust to life with daily-wear contact lenses. Sometimes a willing friend or relative helps with the lens care and handling. Aphakes also have some distinct advantages to mitigate their particular problems when it comes to contact lens wear. Since the cornea has been cut (and nerves severed) during the cataract extraction, the eyes are less sensitive and contact lenses feel more comfortable. (Unfortunately this desensitization may mean that the aphake is less aware of any injury and damage to the eyes; therefore these patients require careful monitoring.) For those who can't cope, there are two more alternatives: extended-wear contact lenses, and intraocular lenses.

Extended-Wear Contact Lenses. As discussed previously this is a recent development, and many eye practitioners feel that these lenses are the safest alternative. As such they have become the single most frequently prescribed form of contact lenses for aphakes. And with good reason: extended-wear contact lenses are comfortable and provide good visual acuity. Primarily they solve the biggest drawback of aphakic contact lens wear by eliminating the daily insertion, removal, and cleaning required of all other types of contact lenses. In fact, extended wear for aphakes was FDA approved before extended wear for so-called "cosmetic" use because of the very real and greater need for this type of lens.

Extended-wear contact lenses are initially inserted at the doctor's office and worn continuously for up to one month or more. During periodic eye examinations at the doctor's office the lenses are usually removed and cleaned and then reinserted. As with daily-wear lenses, sometimes a neighbor or a relative is enlisted to help remove, clean, and insert the lenses between office visits.

Extended wear does have its drawbacks (see Chapter Six for more information). The lenses currently available will not fit everyone, but they are successful in an estimated 75 percent of the aphakic population. Since they wear them for longer periods of time, aphakes tend to have even more of a problem with protein deposits than normally occurs with the daily-wear lenses. The useful life of the lens is thus shorter, necessitating frequent replacement, though the "saline eyewash" (see pp. 132–33) has been shown to be an effective preventive that can be used without removing the lens. Wearers should be hygiene conscious and be willing to go to the doctor for the needed follow-up visits.

Intraocular Lenses. Although they are not contact lenses, plastic intraocular lenses are quite similar and offer a viable and permanent solution for the aphake. Each year a larger percentage of those who undergo cataract removal will have a lens implant, usually at the time of cataract surgery. As a result they have a new substitute lens built right into the eye; quite often vision is restored to 20/20 without glasses. This is the most convenient form of cataract correction, since the lens is never removed unless complications ensue.

The intraocular lens is the brainchild of the English ophthalmologist Harold Ridley, who developed the idea during World War II. He saw wounded RAF pilots with fragments of Plexiglas windshields embedded in their eyes. The plastic remained inert, which led him to the conclusion that intraocular lenses could be made from the same material (polymethylmethacrylate, or PMMA, the same plastic from which conventional hard contact lenses are made) and safely placed into the eye. He implanted the first such lens in 1949.

Since ophthalmologists do not know the long-term effects of intraocular lens implants, the best candidates for ocular implants are the elderly. If they have dry eyes and eyelid abnormalities, which preclude wearing contact lenses, the lens implant will be the best type of vision correction. On the other hand those who are very nearsighted, have detached retinas, poorly controlled glaucoma, diabetes, or other eye diseases, are advised to seek the other vision-corrective devices mentioned earlier.

About 10 percent of the intraocular implants result in com-

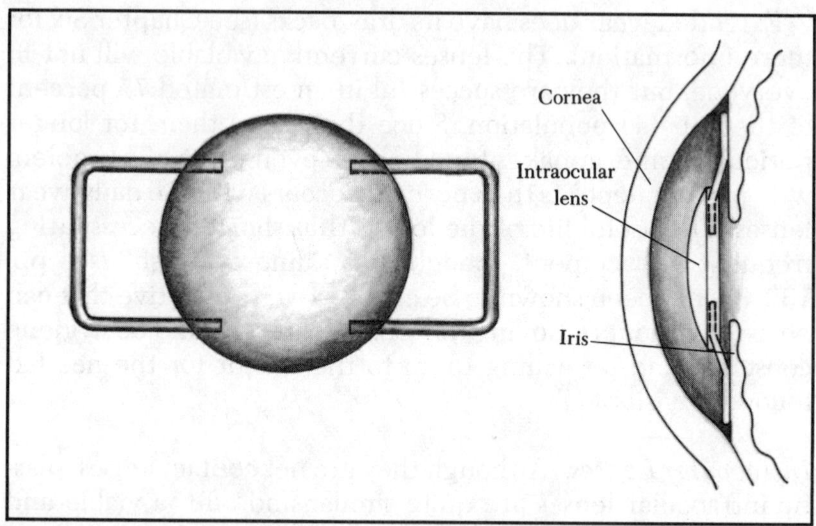

Figure 28. Intraocular lens.

plications. Many of these can be corrected without removing the implant. They may include dislocation of the implant, changes in the cornea, inflammation of the iris, retinal detachment, and increased pressure in the eye that could lead to glaucoma. At times the intraocular lens will have to be removed. Tests are still being conducted to study the long-term effects of intraocular lenses.

Future developments in this field lie mainly in the improvement of the lenses themselves. Another method of vision correction involves grafting "live" contact lenses onto the aphake's cornea. Donor corneas are frozen and ground to size, then sutured onto the living host cornea. To date several such operations have been successful.

THE X-CHROM LENS FOR COLOR BLINDNESS

It is estimated that there are 8.5 million people in the United States who have some degree of *color blindness.* This is the common name given to the inability to distinguish colors and shades; some people have trouble with only a few colors, others see no colors at all. This inherited disorder affects mostly males: 8 percent of the male population is red-green color deficient, as compared with only one half of 1 percent of the female population.

Eye practitioners can test you if you suspect you are color deficient. Telltale signs include a lack of interest in colors, choosing color combinations that don't appeal to most people, a preference toward blues and yellows and indifference toward reds and greens, unawareness of fall foliage, difficulty in seeing veins and freckles, and the preference of black-and-white TV over color.

In the past there was nothing available to improve color blindness. But several years ago Dr. Harry Zeltzer developed a special, red-tinted contact lens that improves the color perception of those who suffer the most common type of color blindness (red-green). (A red-tinted lens in eyeglasses doesn't work because the lens is too far away from the eye.) The X-Chrom lens has been a godsend to people whose jobs and interests require the ability to identify colors. Telephone repairmen, hunters, drivers, home handymen, painters, cosmeticians, printers, textile workers, chemists, photographers, artists, decorators, and anyone who selects clothes (even if it's just their own)—all can benefit from this type of lens. It has even helped color-deficient children who were wrongly labeled as learning deficient.

The X-Chrom lens is deep red in color. Only one tinted lens is prescribed, usually for the nondominant eye. It works by changing the relative intensities of red and green objects. The nondominant (corrected) eye supplies the brain with information about colors that are normally hard for it to identify; the dominant (uncorrected) eye continues to supply the colors the eye is capable of seeing correctly. As if by magic the wearer sees colors he never even knew existed. At first colors may seem to glow or be more vibrant, and objects that used to blend into the background may seem to jump out. But the eye and brain soon adjust to the unfamiliar information: the newly perceived colors are identified and learned.

If necessary the X-Chrom lens can be manufactured to incorporate a prescription to correct refractive errors. In that case the wearer keeps his regular clear lens in the dominant eye and the X-Chrom corrective lens in the other. Usually a third, clear contact lens incorporating the necessary prescription is kept on hand for use in the nondominant eye when the

X-Chrom is not worn. Those who do not wish to wear a contact lens in both eyes can wear glasses over the X-Chrom lens.

The fitting, adjustment period, wearing, care, and handling of the lens are the same as for conventional hard lenses, but the cost is higher. The X-Chrom may be worn during both daytime and nighttime, but many elect to remove the lens at night because of the reduced illumination that will be exaggerated with this lens. Some wearers experience a slight reduction in visual acuity, or their depth perception is affected because the two eyes receive unequal amounts of illumination. Cosmetically the red color of the X-Chrom lens is very obvious. All these disadvantages must be weighed against enhanced color perception. The color-blind patient, therefore, has to be well motivated in order to wear this lens.

Clearly the X-Chrom offers no guarantees and is not for every color-deficient patient. In the words of its developer it's "an aid, not a cure." But for most color-blind people it means improved color perception and opens up new vistas in everyday pleasures and work.

CONTACT LENSES FOR KERATOCONUS

Keratoconus is a relatively common hereditary disorder that manifests itself in adolescence. It affects both eyes, but one eye usually progresses faster than the other. During the course of this disease the cornea changes from its round shape to that of a cone, hence the name: *kera* meaning "cornea" and *conus* meaning "cone." The apex of the cone is thin and may become scarred. In severe cases the apex may actually perforate.

The poor vision brought on by keratoconus is due to a highly exaggerated form of astigmatism that is poorly corrected by glasses. Until contact lenses became available, keratoconus patients often had to be satisfied with partially corrected vision and led less-than-normal lives. But contact lenses can provide almost perfect vision in most cases and are the best means of vision correction for this disorder.

Hard contact lenses are usually used because the smooth, dome-shaped shell plus the tears beneath it provide a new smooth, round refracting surface for the eye. Because the cornea is diseased, the eye may not tolerate conventional hard lenses. In that case gas-permeable contact lenses (see Chapter

Five) may be prescribed instead. Soft contact lenses, in general, do not work well with keratoconic eyes. As is the case with astigmatism, the pliable material from which they are made conforms to the misshapen cornea, duplicating the refractive error. Soft contact lenses may, however, correct a portion of the faulty vision. And in some cases the patient is fitted with hard lenses on top of the soft lenses, piggyback fashion, to take advantage of the comfort of the soft lens plus the sharp visual acuity provided by the hard lens. In all cases the lenses are difficult to manufacture, and the fitting process must be extremely exact to achieve acceptable results.

COSMETIC AND PROSTHETIC CONTACT LENSES

PROSTHETIC CONTACT LENSES

This type of lens has been put to artistic use in the movies by actors creating bizarre special effects, such as the eyes of monsters. Ironically prosthetic lenses can also be of real help to those who need something special in order to appear normal. They can dramatically improve the appearance (and sometimes the vision as well) of eyes that have been disfigured or in some way appear abnormal. This includes those who suffer from albinism or unsightly, deformed eyes whose defect is congenital in origin or due to accidental injury or a result of eye surgery. The ultimate type of prosthetic contact lens is the one that forms the "false eye"—or shell over the entire socket when an eye is enucleated (surgically removed).

Prosthetic contact lenses, which may cover the entire sclera or only the cornea, are predominantly manufactured in rigid form, though soft prosthetic lenses are available. The lenses simulate a normal iris and pupil by incorporating an opaque area that is colored artistically to achieve the final appearance of the eye. The desired image may be placed on any portion of the lens, and may be of any color. It is stable and nontoxic because in one type the image is "painted" on the surface of one lens and then covered with another lens, forming a "sandwich." Another method employs a special tinting process of a soft lens.

COSMETIC CONTACT LENSES

For those who wish to change the color of their eyes, especially actors or models, the cosmetic contact lens is a real boon. Some of these lenses cover only the cornea, are made of rigid PMMA material, and are opaque, except in the transparent central area. This clear zone covers the pupil and may have a prescription incorporated. Obviously the lens has to center perfectly. Fitting is difficult and may require many sessions. Care and handling is similar to the standard hard lens. Soft lenses may also be tinted to provide similar cosmetic results.

ORTHOKERATOLOGY

The term *orthokeratology* comes from the words *ortho,* meaning "straight," and *keratology,* relating to the cornea. It should come as no surprise then that this form of vision therapy seeks to actually change the curvature of the cornea—in order to lessen the refractive error. Using much the same principle as an orthodontist employs when using braces to correct the position of wayward teeth, orthokeratology utilizes a series of relatively flat, hard PMMA contact lenses to mold the cornea gradually into the desired shape.

The process is a long and costly one. The success rate is quite low, the process may be very uncomfortable, and there are no guarantees. Even when successful the result is fleeting unless "retainer" lenses are worn periodically to prevent the elastic cornea from "bouncing back" to its natural shape. Most ophthalmologists object to this practice, citing the inadvisability of altering such a sensitive part of the anatomy (especially when so many safer alternatives are available.) There is also the possibility of permanently damaging the cornea. Nevertheless orthokeratology does have its advocates, and experimentation and research continue.

SURGERY AS A MEANS TO CORRECT REFRACTIVE ERRORS

There are three methods, highly controversial and still experimental, that can correct errors of refraction:

RADIAL KERATOTOMY

This surgical procedure may be performed on those nearsighted people who cannot or do not wish to wear eyeglasses

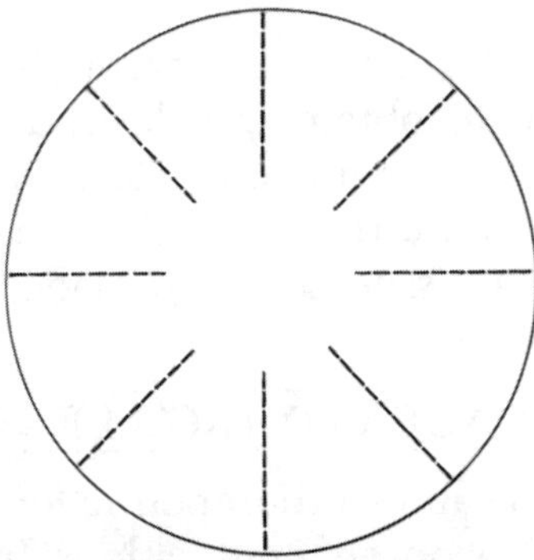

Figure 29. Radial keratotomy.

or contact lenses. The process consists of making a series of eight to sixteen radial incisions in the cornea, much like the spokes of a wheel. The incisions are about half the thickness of the cornea, and do not meet in the center, thus sparing the pupillary zone. The scored cornea flattens in shape as the incisions heal, a process that takes approximately six to eight weeks. The result is a reduction of myopia. Each patient undergoing this procedure has to be carefully selected as to degree of myopia and the thickness and condition of the cornea. Like other forms of surgery, radial keratotomy cannot be guaranteed, and complications such as scarring and perforations in the cornea can occur. The surgery can be performed as an outpatient procedure under local anesthesia. The average cost is two thousand dollars. A national investigational study is under way to determine the efficacy of radial keratotomy.

KERATOPHAKIA

Only aphakia and hyperopia can be corrected using this method, which involves the use of a human corneal donor button. The donor cornea is frozen and lathe-cut and shaped by computer technology. A portion of the recipient cornea is removed surgically and the donor button is sutured onto or placed in a center pocket of the recipient cornea. The resultant combination corrects the refractive error.

KERATOMILEUSIS

Still another experimental surgical technique utilizes a vibrating microkeratome (tiny surgical knife), which removes a 1-mm-thick slice from the patient's cornea. The slice is promptly frozen and a computer-controlled cryolathe fashions the underside of the slice to obtain the desired correction of the refractive error. After thawing out, the newly shaped corneal slice is sutured back onto the patient's cornea. In essence the patient's own corneal tissue has been made into a permanent contact lens.

BANDAGE CONTACT LENSES

A bandage lens, also called a therapeutic lens, is a special soft, very thin, high-water-content contact lens. In 1974 this hydrophilic lens was the first type to be used on an extended-wear basis, but without incorporating a prescription. It has a wide variety of uses before ocular surgery, after ocular surgery, and sometimes instead of surgery. It can also be therapeutic in conditions that do not respond to any other form of treatment.

The lens functions basically as a protective shield and prevents a damaged or ailing cornea from coming into contact with the eyelids and the air. Healing is thereby accelerated and pain is alleviated for as long as the lens is worn, which is on an extended basis (more than twenty-four hours). As such it can take the place of the tight eyepatch formerly used to immobilize the eye to facilitate the recovery process. It is usually needed only temporarily until the condition being treated has cleared up. The lens is placed on the cornea by the ophthalmologist and is removed by the doctor when the disorder being treated has been cured.

USES OF BANDAGE LENSES

The lens has been used for many years with varying degrees of success to treat a great number of conditions. The most frequent uses are for:

Dry Eyes. Although I have cautioned against the use of a soft lens when tear production is reduced, this lens plays an important role in severe cases of dry eyes. The dry-eye syndrome is a common by-product of the aging process and affects women more often than men. In postmenopausal women all the mucous membranes begin to dry because of the shift in hormone production. In these cases dryness of the eye can become quite severe. A dry eye may also be caused by drugs (birth control pills, antihistamines, and so on), injury to or infection of the lachrymal glands, autoimmune disorders (Stevens-Johnson syndrome), severe injuries or infections of the eye, and vitamin deficiencies.

Eyes with a marked reduction in tear production can lead to damaged corneas. For patients suffering from dry eyes a bandage lens in tandem with *frequent instillation of artificial tears* is an excellent treatment. The eye drops are absorbed by the highly hydrophilic (water-loving) lens, bathing the eye with them in a more constant fashion than if drops alone were used.

Bullous Keratopathy. As a result of the aging process or following injury to the eye, which may be accidental or occur after intraocular surgery such as cataract extraction, the cornea may swell with an abnormal amount of fluid. The inner surface of the cornea *(endothelium)* becomes damaged, vision becomes blurred, and there is marked pain. The bandage lens can reduce and sometimes completely alleviate both symptoms by protecting the eroded corneal surface and by acting as a barrier to prevent fluid from escaping from the cornea.

Corneal Ulcers and Abrasions. The bandage lens seems to accelerate the healing process in abrasions and ulcers that can result from viral, bacterial, and fungal infections. This form of treatment should only be used in conjunction with antibiotic, antiviral, or antifungal eye drops.

Trichiasis. As a result of an injury, infection, or aging, the eyelashes may turn inward and rub against the cornea. A bandage lens can act as a shield while (or until) the primary condition is treated.

Chemical and Thermal Burns. By eliminating the constant irritation of the eyelid coming into contact with the healing corneal tissue, a bandage lens allows the cornea to grow back normally and more rapidly. Using a bandage lens postoperatively after a burn increases the success rate of such surgery.

Penetrating Corneal Wounds. When the cornea becomes

wounded, a bandage lens aids in forming a protective shield and can be employed to facilitate healing when surgery has to be delayed.

Bell's Palsy. When the upper lid is unable to close completely, the cornea may become overly dry. The bandage lens protects the cornea, but frequent instillation of artificial tears is necessary as an adjunct.

THE "CONTACT LENS" AS A DRUG DELIVERY SYSTEM

There now exist tiny discs containing special medication that may be placed on the eye to provide a constant source of medication. The small oval-shaped flexible "lens" is worn over the sclera under the eyelid. Its sole purpose is to act as a reservoir for drugs in liquid form, allowing specific amounts to be released into the eye gradually over a prolonged period of time. It's really a time-release capsule for the eyes. The drug in use is, therefore, more effective than when it is administered as intermittent drops, because constant, round-the-clock treatment is possible. Also lesser amounts of the drug may do the job with this method. This can in turn reduce the local and systemic side effects and allow the use of more potent drugs such as steroids and glaucoma medication. Once in place the "contact lens" is a convenient way of administering medication, particularly for patients who might not otherwise comply with the prescribed treatment. Ocusert™, containing the glaucoma medication pilocarpine, and Lacrisert™, containing lubricating medication, are the two special "lenses" now commercially available. They can be worn continuously (even while sleeping) and removed and replaced weekly for the duration of the treatment.

CHAPTER EIGHT

CONTACT LENS PROBLEMS AND HOW TO SOLVE THEM

NORMAL SYMPTOMS WHILE WEARING CONTACT LENSES

During the adaptation period, and especially during the first two days, there are several symptoms you can expect to encounter. This adaptation period largely involves the adjustment of the cornea to the new lens; in addition there are many other subtle adjustments that you will automatically begin to make as you gradually learn to live with this new optical device. These symptoms, which are more common with hard lenses than with soft, merely mean that your eyes are reacting to the presence of "foreign bodies" (the contact lenses). Such reactions are quite normal and no cause for alarm. Your eyes will eventually learn to tolerate the presence of these foreign bodies, and the symptoms will disappear. If any of the following symptoms become severe, or if you feel any real pain while wearing the lenses, be sure to consult your eye doctor.

- *Difficulty gazing upward.* Due to the edge of the eyelid bumping into the upper edge of the lens.

- *Light sensitivity.* Due to mild irritation of the cornea.

- *Frequent blinking.* Due to the presence of a foreign-body sensation.

- *Watery, teary eyes.* Due to the presence of a foreign-body sensation.

• *"Flare."* Reflections of light caused by poor centering of lenses.

• *Mild redness, itching, and burning.* Due to dryness or pollution of the air, especially indoors where the air may be dry and/or smoke filled.

• *Mildly blurred vision.* Due to increased tearing, a poorly centered lens, or a dry lens.

• *Displaced lens.* Due to excessive tearing; lenses may move off center, or slide under the eyelids. (See pp. 71–73 and 108–10 for recentering lenses.)

• *Tired eyes.* Due to the slight strain of the adaptation period.

• *Squinting.* Due to light sensitivity or blurred vision.

ABNORMAL SYMPTOMS

The following symptoms are more serious. If any occur to you, remove your lenses immediately and notify your eye doctor. Those marked with an asterisk (*) may occur in mild form during the adaptation period, and are no cause for alarm.

SYMPTOM	CAUSE	CURE
*Blurred vision with lenses on	Wrong lens power	New lens prescription; modify present lens (for hard lenses).
	Poorly fitted lens causing bubbles, edema, off-center position on eye	New lens prescription; modify present lens (for hard lenses).
	*Tearing	Adaptation
	Deposits on lens surfaces (makeup, mucus, etc.)	Clean lenses well at home; use enzyme solution (for soft lenses); send to your doctor for thorough professional cleaning.
	Switched lenses	Reverse lenses; if unsure, have practitioner check lenses; put dot on right lens (if hard contacts) to prevent future mixups; maintain a routine, starting with the right lens first.

SYMPTOM	CAUSE	CURE
	Scratches	Send to lab for polishing (if hard lens); soft lenses, and hard lenses with deep scratches, require a new lens.
*Blurry vision after lenses are removed ("spectacle blur")	Edema—swollen cornea due to oxygen deprivation usually after an excessively prolonged wearing time	Shorten wearing time; new or modified lenses (fenestrations, smaller or thinner lenses, gas-permeable, or soft lenses); blinking exercises.
	Corneal abrasion	Shorten wearing time; new lens prescription or modify present lenses; verify that you are inserting, removing, and centering your lenses properly.
	Corneal molding from poorly fitted lenses (hard lenses)	New lens prescription or modify fit of present lenses; switch to soft or gas-permeable lenses. For corneal abrasion consult your ophthalmologist.
*Burning sensation	Dry eyes	Relieve condition with frequent use of artificial tears; change working environment; install a humidifier; cease use of certain drugs such as birth control pills, or antihistamines; pregnancy and menopause may also cause hormonal changes and dry eyes; occasionally lens wear must be discontinued.
Pain after removing lenses (usually at night)	Overwear syndrome, leading to oxygen deprivation and corneal edema (swelling)	Take aspirin; apply cold compress for immediate relief. Depending on the severity of the case, recovery may occur within hours or several days. To prevent recurrence shorten wearing time or switch to gas-permeable or soft lenses; hard lenses may be modified with fenestrations.
	Corneal abrasion	Consult your ophthalmologist.
Pain while wearing lens	Foreign object under lens; damaged lens	Remove and inspect lens for dirt or damage; if dirty, clean lens and reinsert; if nicked or scratched, report to practitioner.
*Sensitivity to light while wearing lenses	Corneal irritation, overwear syndrome, or improperly fitted lens	Shorten wearing schedule; have practitioner check lens fit; may have to switch to thinner, fenestrated, gas-permeable, or soft lenses. Wear sunglasses.

SYMPTOM	CAUSE	CURE
*Excessive tearing	Poor-quality lenses; badly fitted lenses	Have practitioner examine eyes and check fit; new lens prescriptions or polish edges of present hard lenses.
	Foreign body under lens; damaged lens	Remove and inspect lens for dirt or damage; if dirty, clean and reinsert lens; if damaged, notify practitioner.
*"Flare," usually at night with hard lenses	Larger pupil picks up light reflecting off lens edge	Larger diameter lenses.
*Scratchy feeling	Rough lens edges	Send hard lens to doctor for polishing.
	Deposits on lenses	Clean soft lens with enzyme solution.
	Dry eyes	See "Burning sensation."
*Itchiness	Allergic reaction to chemicals in solutions used for soft lenses	Switch to unpreserved saline solutions and heat disinfection.
	Systemic allergy	Treat allergy with antihistamines; if symptoms persist, lens wear may have to cease temporarily.
	Dry eyes	See "Burning sensation."
Halos around lights	Corneal edema due to overwear syndrome	Increase tear exchange by modifying lens fit and/or fenestrations; switch to thinner, smaller lenses, or to gas-permeable or soft lenses; shorten wearing time.
*Bubbles under lens	Poor lens fit	New lens prescription or modify present hard lens.
*Redness	Overwear syndrome	See "Pain after removing lenses."
	Allergy to solutions or systemic allergy	See "Itchiness."
	Infection (conjunctivitis)	Remove lenses; doctor will prescribe topical antibiotic in the form of eye drops.
Mucus or discharge	Allergic reaction to solutions or systemic allergy	See "Itchiness."
	Infection (conjunctivitis)	See "Redness."

CONTACT LENS EMERGENCIES

A contact lens doesn't always behave the way you expect it to. The following situations may be alarming, unless you know how to deal with them. If you have any doubts or problems, be sure to consult your eye doctor.

ALL TYPES OF LENSES

Right and Left Lenses Mixed Up:	Check vision in each eye individually by covering the other eye with your hand. If vision in the uncovered eye seems blurry, or if lenses are uncomfortable, switch lenses. If this happens often and you have hard lenses, your doctor can mark the right one with an identifying dot to prevent future mixups.
The Lens Is Displaced on Your Eye:	Locate the lens and recenter it as directed on pages 71–73 for hard lenses or pages 108–10 for soft lenses.
The Lens Is Damaged:	A hard lens may crack or chip; a soft lens may tear. *Never insert a damaged lens.* Put it in the case and return it to your practitioner for a replacement.
Dropped Lens:	The first rule is *don't move.* Remove your shoes to safeguard against crushing the lens. Look all around the ground near you (or have someone else do this for you). Don't neglect inspecting your clothing. (One soft contact lens wearer dropped her lens in the bathroom. Two days later she found it shriveled up like a cornflake but miraculously undamaged, on the kitchen floor. The lens had obviously hitched a ride on her clothing. When hydrated with saline the lens returned to its normal state.) So if at first you don't succeed, keep looking. If indoors you can focus a flashlight in the direction the lens is likely to have fallen; its shiny

surface will be highlighted. Once you find the lens, don't slide it along the ground. Pick it up by touching it with a moistened fingertip (not saliva) to which it will stick. If it's landed dome side up, it probably won't cling to your fingertip because of the suction created. In this case sprinkle a few drops of water over it to loosen its grip; then slide a piece of paper under it and scoop it up.

(Needless to say, if you insert contact lenses over a sink, you should make certain that the stopper is in place, or that there's a paper towel over the drain. If not you may end up with 20/20 plumbing. Sometimes playing—or paying—the plumber produces a lost lens. More often it just creates a mess.)

Always clean the lens before reinserting it. Soft lenses should be cleaned, disinfected, and rehydrated. Inspect the lens carefully for damage and if you suspect there's any, have your contact lens specialist inspect it.

HARD LENSES AND CAS PERMEABLE LENSES

Lens Stuck Under Upper Eyelid:	Place your head back, open your eye, and flood the eye with cool tap water until the lens moves freely.
Lens Stuck on White of Eye:	Flood the eye with cool tap water until the suction is broken and the lens can be recentered and then removed. You may also use a suction removal device, available from your eye doctor.
Foreign Body Under Lens:	This can be quite painful, necessitating immediate removal of the lens. Put the lens in its carrying case until you can clean it and reinsert it as usual. *Do not pop it into your mouth.*

SOFT LENSES AND EXTENDED-WEAR LENSES	
Lens Cannot Be Unfolded:	Allow the lens to soak in saline solution for 10 minutes. Gently rub the lens between your thumb and forefinger until it gradually opens. Check the lens for damage before inserting.
Lens Is Folded on the Eye:	Remove the lens and follow the procedure described above. Never wear a folded lens.
Lens Has Dried in the Case:	Do not touch the lens. Refill the case with saline solution and wait 10 minutes for the lens to rehydrate. When it has regained its suppleness and transparency, it will be as good as new. (Make sure you check it, though, for possible damage.)
Lens Is Stuck to Your Eye:	You probably forgot to add the salt tablet to the distilled water. Do not try to remove the lens. Remix some saline solution and put a few drops directly into your eye to loosen the lens and return it to its normal fitting characteristics. You may then remove it as usual.

CHAPTER NINE

QUESTIONS AND ANSWERS

These are the questions asked most frequently by my patients. If you have any others (not covered in the text of this book), consult your contact lens specialist.

Q: *Can the eye become dependent on contact lenses?*
A: No. Wearing contact lenses neither improves nor worsens vision. The only "dependence" is a psychological one. The excellent vision correction provided, the convenience, and the improvement of one's appearance make many wearers contact lens "addicts."

Q: *Why is my vision blurry while wearing eyeglasses after I remove my contact lenses?*
A: This condition is called *spectacle blur.* It usually occurs with hard lenses and is due to corneal molding. The cornea is pliable and its shape is changed slightly by the contact lens, much as the skin of your finger becomes indented by a ring. Just as the indentation on your finger disappears after the ring is removed, your cornea gradually assumes its original shape. In the meantime you have an irregularly curved cornea causing a kind of "induced astigmatism," for which your spectacles were not ground to correct. As a result of this temporary and artificial refractive error your vision is slightly blurry when you switch to spectacles. This situation may last from a few minutes to a few hours.

Q: *Why do I see differently when I switch back to glasses?*
A: See discussion of spectacle blur. Also this difference in vi-

sion may be due to the fact that spectacles for nearsightedness reduce the size of objects and those for farsightedness magnify objects (especially for aphakics, who are very farsighted). With contact lenses there is no such effect. When you switch from contacts to glasses, your brain becomes momentarily confused and interprets the smaller or larger image as blurry. Again this phenomenon is fleeting and only mildly annoying if you wear contacts most of your waking hours. Should you decide to return to full-time spectacle wear, your brain will adapt to this different way of seeing in a short period of time.

Q: *Why can't I use saliva to clean contact lenses?*
A: Though the composition of saliva makes it a very efficacious wetting solution for hard lenses, it is absolutely unacceptable to use it for this purpose. Saliva contains bacteria (and possibly viruses and fungi) that are safe for the mouth, but dangerous for the eye.

Q: *Can I use hard contact lens solutions for soft lenses and vice versa?*
A: Absolutely not. These solutions were designed for specific types of plastic. Because hard lenses and soft lenses have very different properties, their accompanying solutions contain different ingredients. In addition soft lenses will absorb the chemicals in the hard-lens solutions; these chemicals can later be released into the eye, possibly causing irritation or ocular damage.

Q: *Can contact lenses be used in sports?*
A: The bony structure (orbit) that forms the eye socket was designed to protect you from injury, and it does its job extremely well. But if you're very active in sports, for instance, hard lenses may pose problems. If you are hit directly in the eye with a racquet ball, wearing a hard contact might result in greater ocular injury than if you were not wearing lenses. That a contact lens would shatter, however, is highly unlikely: the plastic from which it is made requires the force of a hammer striking it on a cement surface in order to break it. Of course, soft lenses are safer. In some instances a contact lens can actually act as a barrier and shield the eye from scratches. However, for contact sports and racquet sports you should wear

special protective glasses, goggles, or masks, whether you wear contact lenses or not.

Q: *Can contact lenses harm the eye?*
A: Contact lenses are dangerous if you have a faulty lens, or do not maintain proper ocular hygiene, or don't follow the recommended wearing and handling procedures. For instance, *corneal abrasion* can occur when the lens isn't inserted properly. *Corneal edema* occurs if you overwear the lens. An eye infection may be caused by fingers or contact lens solutions that are contaminated. And foreign bodies can sneak under the lens and irritate the cornea.

With regard to the vast number of contact lens wearers, though, such complications have been remarkably rare.

Q: *What is corneal edema?*
A: It is the most common contact lens complication and the main reason you can't wear lenses for twenty-four hours (except for extended-wear contacts). Edema means swelling, which is what happens to your cornea when you wear your lenses too long and deprive the cornea of oxygen. Even though gas-permeable lenses, soft lenses, and lenses that allow optimum tear exchange reduce the chance of edema, there is always less oxygen than normally reaches the naked eye. You'll know when you've been wearing your contacts too long: your eyes will burn, turn red, be light sensitive; maybe you'll see halos or rainbows around lights. Unless you're too stubborn or highly motivated, the most appealing thought in the world will be that of removing your lenses, which is exactly the right thing to do. In minor cases your cornea will recuperate in a few hours (better yet—overnight). If you really overdo it, recovery may take several days and corneal abrasion may follow.

Q: *What is conjunctivitis?*
A: This is an infection of the conjunctiva, the mucous membrane that covers the white part of the eye and lines the underside of the eyelids. Conjunctivitis and other eye infections can afflict the contact lens wearer who doesn't clean (and disinfect, in the case of soft lenses) his lenses according to instructions. It can also occur when wearers clean and wet the lenses with saliva, which is loaded with bacteria, viruses, and perhaps

fungi. In addition to the ordinary garden-variety conjunctivitis ("pink eye"), there's another form called "giant papillary conjunctivitis," which is caused only by contact lens wear (the contact lenses themselves, deposits on the lenses, or any of the contact lens solutions). In treating the individual with this type of conjunctivitis I discard the contact lens and prescribe a steroid (cortisone) eye drop. Resolution of the disorder may take days or even weeks. Once the conjunctiva has healed, I order a new lens and then instruct the patient to use different solutions. For the hard contact lens wearer the correct solution is determined by trial and error. For the soft contact lens wearer I permit only the use of unpreserved saline and the heat method of disinfection. Happily, this type of conjunctivitis, when treated properly, rarely recurs. If it does reappear, cessation of contact lens use may be the only solution.

Q: *What's corneal abrasion?*
A: Corneal abrasion is the term used when the surface layer of the cornea is scraped or scratched off. This can occur when you wear the contact lenses too long (overwear syndrome); with improperly fitted lenses; or by inserting, removing, or recentering the lens improperly. Sleeping with daily-wear lenses on often leads to corneal abrasion. The symptoms are decreased vision, burning pain, sensitivity to light, the sensation of having something in your eye, and copious tearing. Abrasion that follows corneal edema may not be evident until hours after the contact lenses have been removed. Healing is mercifully rapid: usually within thirty-six hours. You may take aspirin for the pain, and cold compresses may help. Consult your ophthalmologist to make sure there are no complications; he may also recommend that you wear a tight eye patch for the duration of the recuperative period to keep the eye immobile. Though most cases of corneal abrasion are minor, a severe infection can invade the damaged cells. While this is unlikely to occur, it is a possibility, so don't treat corneal abrasions lightly.

Q: *Can contact lenses cause drooping of the eyelids?*
A: It's rare, but the results of one study indicate that in a very few cases, contact lens wear can lead to a condition called *blepharoptosis,* resulting in eyelids that appear to droop. All the patients studied had been wearing hard lenses, some for

many years. The researchers' most likely explanation is that the condition was caused by excessive manipulation and rubbing of the eyelids, usually because of difficulties in inserting and removing the lenses. The trauma caused eyelid muscle damage. This condition can be corrected surgically.

Q: *Why is it harmful to rub the eyes while wearing contact lenses, even soft ones?*
A: There are several reasons: (1) Because of the aforementioned blepharoptosis, (2) because an abrasion may occur, and (3) because of the possible introduction of bacteria, fungi, or viruses.

Q: *How many hours a day can I expect to wear contact lenses?*
A: That depends upon the lens and your eyes. Most people are eventually able to wear their lenses most of their waking hours: about eight hours for hard-lens wearers and fourteen hours for soft-lens wearers. But every pair of eyes is unique. Some people can wear their lenses for only four hours a day; some can go for as long as eighteen hours, though this is not a good idea unless you break up the time with a rest period. This method can be used by anyone to effectively extend wearing time: Remove your lenses and let the eyes rest for fifteen or twenty minutes. This gives them a new lease on life, and lets you wear your lenses late at night after a long day at the office.

Q: *But what if I want to wear contacts just for special occasions?*
A: This can only be done if you wear soft lenses or gas-permeable lenses. Once you've adapted to hard lenses, you should wear them every day for the same number of hours. Otherwise the eye will "unadapt" and the lenses will become uncomfortable. Soft and gas-permeable lenses are less demanding where adaptation is concerned, and you can safely and comfortably wear them intermittently—for the weekend softball game, your triweekly jog, or just for social events.

Q: *Is there an age barrier in contact lens wear?*
A: Theoretically speaking, no. I have fitted infants and ninety-year-olds with contact lenses, and every age in between. One of my patients is in her seventies and has been wearing contact lenses since the 1940s . . . a true pioneer! Infants wear contact lenses not out of vanity, but for therapeutic visual reasons.

Teen-agers adapt to contact lenses very quickly, a testimony to the importance of motivation and the role that improved appearance plays in successful contact lens wear. Puberty may herald marked changes in refractive errors; therefore these youngsters should be examined at least twice a year.

Though contact lenses can be worn at any age, eager parents should wait until a child is ready to use them. The child should be motivated, versed in hygiene, mature enough to accept the responsibility for caring for the lenses, and have the necessary motor skills for handling these tiny, delicate lenses. This usually occurs around the age of twelve. In certain cases parents may be taught to insert and remove the lenses for those too young to have the manual dexterity to do so themselves.

Q: *If my prescription seems to change frequently, can I still wear contact lenses? Won't it be more expensive than changing the prescription of my eyeglasses?*
A: Unless a medical contraindication exists, there is no reason you cannot wear contact lenses—even if the prescription changes frequently. The cost of the new contact lenses usually is comparable to that of new spectacle lenses. In fact changes of spectacles may prove to be the more expensive of the two.

Q: *Is there some magic formula for being able to wear contact lenses successfully?*
A: Yes, in a way. And there are three ingredients:

1. The eye practitioner. Select an expert eye practitioner who specializes in contact lenses. An ophthalmologist or optometrist in private practice is your best choice. With proper medical care, you'll be most likely to wear your contact lenses comfortably and without damaging your eyes. Don't forget: you get what you pay for. Unfortunately there are a multitude of unhappy contact lens wearers who bought "bargain lenses" and then discovered that they were no bargain at all.

2. Motivation. Depending upon the type of lens and your own unique physiology, contact lens wear brings some initial discomfort. You must be sufficiently motivated to tolerate this initial adaptation period, as well as any little difficulties that may crop up later.

3. *Follow instructions!* Many unsuccessful contact lens wearers simply didn't take care of their lenses and eyes properly. The result is reduced lens life, wearing discomfort, poor vision, and possible eye injury.

Q: *What are the most common reasons that contact lens wearers give up their lenses?*
A: There are very few failures if the three above-stated rules are followed. However, the occasionally unsuccessful hard-lens wearer fails most often because of a higher-than-average sensitivity to a foreign-body sensation in the eye. Soft-lens wearers sometimes have an allergic sensitivity to the chemicals used to sterilize the contacts. Other reasons include less-than-perfect vision, frustration with the care and handling of contact lenses, a reduced wearing time, and spectacle blur. But these hindrances, as with almost all contact lens problems, can usually be solved if the eye practitioner is imaginative, skillful, and knowledgeable in the field of contact lenses.

Q: *What advice would you give someone who'd like to wear contacts, but is very afraid of putting something in his eyes?*
A: Fear of wearing contact lenses and especially of inserting the lenses is quite common, but usually disappears with time, patience, and practice. Of course one solution is to prescribe extended-wear contact lenses, which are only removed and inserted every one or two weeks (for general cosmetic wear) and every month or longer for those who have undergone cataract extraction. This is a particularly satisfactory solution for the elderly.

Q: *Do contact lenses slow down or prevent the progression of nearsightedness?*
A: Some eye-care practitioners think it may. However, there is no scientifically accepted proof that this is the case. It's generally believed that heredity determines whether your eyes will require weaker or stronger correction in the future. Contact lenses or glasses have no effect upon the progression of refractive errors.

Q: *Why do my contacts bother me when I read (or study) late at night?*
A: This is a version of the overwear syndrome and is due to a lack of tears and of oxygen to the cornea. When you read, you tend to blink less often. This decreases the tear exchange and your lenses dry out. The cornea doesn't get its quota of oxygen, and mucus may cling to the lens surface. As a result, your eyes may burn, become red, and feel painful, and your vision will not be as sharp as you'd like. This can also occur when your vision is fixed on a relatively nearby object for any length of time, such as watching TV. The solution is to force yourself to blink more frequently or to instill lubricating eye drops.

Q: *Why are my contact lenses a little uncomfortable in the morning?*
A: It could be because you've worn your lenses too long the night before. More commonly, this occurs simply because your eyes aren't yet "awake" and fully functioning. Upon awakening, the eyes are drier than at any other time of the day. Usually if you perform your morning ablutions (showering, shaving, etc.) before inserting your lenses, you give your eyes enough time to prepare them for contact lens insertion. Also you may instill lubricating eye drops upon awakening.

Q: *Why do some people suddenly become unable to wear contact lenses after having worn them for years?*
A: This phenomenon is most common in women, and usually happens in their middle or late twenties. It is suspected that the gradual reduction in tear production ("dry eye") is due to a change in the hormonal balance. Such a hormonal shift is quite frequent in that age group, as it is during or following a pregnancy, following a hysterectomy, while taking birth control pills, or, at a later age, during menopause. The resulting dry eyes can cause the cornea to become oxygen deprived, since there are less oxygen-filled tears.

Symptoms such as decreased comfortable wearing time, a burning sensation, red eyes, and pain suddenly plague those who have been happily wearing lenses for five, ten, or fifteen years. Such an acquired intolerance to contact lenses can also occur to both sexes because of drugs that dry out the eyes. These include tranquilizers, antihistamines, decongestants, diuretics, and those drugs containing belladonna or its derivatives. If you indulge in alcohol or marijuana, your lenses will become uncomfortable because these substances also reduce the amount of tears your eyes produce. A dry environment found in air-conditioned or centrally heated rooms or in a dry climate can have the same effect as well. If you're a frequent flyer, you may notice an increase in discomfort, too, because airplane interiors are notorious for their dry air. *In some cases the eyes have simply lost a tolerance for wearing contact lenses.*

Q: *Do some people have to give up wearing contacts?*
A: Sometimes, as a last resort. But there are many ways to improve the oxygen and tear supply to the cornea. For instance, holes, or fenestrations, can be drilled in hard lenses. You can switch to gas-permeable lenses, to soft lenses, or even to extended-wear lenses. You can use artificial tears (though the necessity of using them frequently can prove to be impractical). You could simply limit the wearing time and learn to live with this. Of course you could also try to alleviate the causes of dry eyes by humidifying your home and office, switching from oral contraceptives to another type, and so on.

Q: *Why shouldn't I wear non–extended-wear contact lenses when I sleep?*
A: Except with extended-wear lenses, sleeping while wearing contact lenses is dangerous because this will deprive your cornea of oxygen. During ordinary wear the lens usually moves with each blink, which allows an exchange of tears to take place. With gas-permeable lenses oxygen also passes through the lens when the eye is open. If the lids remain closed and the lenses remain stationary, as during sleep, the normal corneal metabolism is disturbed. Corneal edema, accompanied by pain, will follow.

Q: *Are there any other times I shouldn't wear contacts?*
A: It's usually best to remove them if you plan to swim, for several reasons. Too much water in your eyes can loosen the lenses and cause them to decenter or fall out. Therefore do not open your eyes more than a crack underwater and stay clear of splashers. Also soft lenses can absorb chemicals and other impurities in the water and become ruined. Salt water will not

harm either hard or soft contact lenses. However, I advise my patients who wish to swim in chlorinated water to remove their contact lenses. (Alternatively, they can wear well-fitted goggles, but these are not effective for everyone. There are prescription goggles available that may interest the very nearsighted.) After leaving the pool, they are instructed to rinse their eyes with plain water; thirty minutes later the contact lenses may be safely reinserted.

It's also a good idea to remove your lenses while showering or shampooing, though some wearers are able to perform this function by shutting their eyes tightly whenever the water approaches their eyes. Be extra wary of getting soap in your eyes. The best solution is to remove the lenses—no easy task mid-shower. You should also keep your contacts out in areas where the air contains hair spray or other irritants. If you have a history of hay fever, you should not wear contacts during the height of the hay fever season.

Q: *Will crying harm my contacts or make them fall out?*
A: A slight crying spell can actually make dry lenses temporarily more comfortable because of the increased tear production. A real gusher, however, could cause contacts—especially hard ones—to become displaced or even to pop out.

Q: *My lenses really bother me when I'm in a smoky room. What can I do?*
A: Not much. You can step outside periodically to give your eyes (as well as your lungs) a breath of fresh air. Artificial tear solutions and lubricating eye drops will help temporarily. Soft-lens wearers should be aware that smoke can be absorbed by their lenses, shortening their useful life.

Q: *I'm planning to take a very long trip, with several stops along the way. If I lose a contact lens, my whole trip will be ruined. What should I do?*
A: Ask your contact lens specialist for the name of a reputable specialist in each area in which you'll be stopping. Make sure you take a copy of your prescription, which includes fitting information. You should consider buying a duplicate pair of contact lenses to take along in case you damage or lose one of the original pair. And bring along your glasses, too—just in case.

Q: *What are the ocular symptoms that indicate I should have my eyes and my contact lenses checked between normally scheduled visits?*
A: There are several subtle signs indicating that your lenses may be due for a reevaluation. If any of these symptoms occur, make an appointment with your doctor for an examination:

- Increased sensation of lenses.
- Reduced wearing time.
- Vision that seems less clear than originally.
- Wearing glasses more and more.
- That feeling that you "can't wait to get your lenses out."

Q: *Can't a contact lens get lost behind the eye?*
A: Absolutely not. If you turn to figure 2, page 5, you'll see that natural anatomical barriers prevent this from happening. A lens can, however, become decentered off the cornea and migrate onto the white of the eye, or get stuck under the eyelid. This is no cause for panic—there are safe and easy methods for returning the contact lens to its rightful place, as explained in the chapters on the various types of lenses.

Q: *Is it true that blue eyes are more sensitive than brown eyes?*
A: It is true that the lighter the pigment in the iris, the less light is filtered and the higher is the intensity of light focused on the retina. Therefore blue eyes are the most light sensitive and brown eyes the least. This is only a minor consideration in contact lens wear, though, since the increase in light sensitivity *(photophobia)* of blue-eyed individuals is minor. Some eyes are more sensitive to foreign bodies (such as contact lenses), but there is no correlation between this type of sensitivity and eye color.

Q: *Can I wear makeup with contacts?*
A: Definitely. It's best, however, to use *water-soluble* products and to stay away from oil-based makeup and makeup removers since oil will fog up the lenses. Water-soluble makeup, on the other hand, will be harmlessly dissolved in the tears. It's also advised that you apply makeup after you've inserted your lenses and to remove the makeup after the lenses are taken out.

Q: *Can I really play sports while wearing contact lenses?*
A: Yes, and better! You can engage in just about any athletic activity, and you'd be surprised at the number of baseball, football, basketball, skiing, hockey, and tennis pros who wear contact lenses (Reggie Jackson and Billie Jean King notwithstanding). Soft contacts are the best for the sports minded, because they don't pop out the way hard lenses do; foreign particles get under them only very rarely, and there is not any danger of them shattering from a hard blow to the eye. In contact sports and racquet sports you should wear some type of protective goggles, glasses, or mask.

Q: *I'm big on snorkeling and scuba diving. Can I wear my lenses while diving?*
A: Yes. Wearing contact lenses has many advantages over other forms of vision correction used with a mask. They don't fog up; they allow for corrected peripheral vision, which adds to the beauty and safety of diving; they allow you to see even on those occasions when you need to remove the mask. For diving, soft contact lenses are preferred over hard because the rigid lenses tend to pop out. Certain precautions should be obeyed, however. First, learn how to close your eyes quickly in case your mask suddenly becomes flooded. Second, don't dive too long or too deeply because there's evidence (from a naval study) that the eyes can suffer from "the bends" and that they may not receive enough oxygen under diving conditions.

Q: *Are there contact lenses that correct cross eyes and other eye muscle disorders?*
A: In certain eye muscle abnormalities such as as cross eyes *(esotropia)* or wall eyes *(exotropia),* a spectacle prescription may help or completely correct the disorder. In these cases contact lenses will provide the same treatment. However, when large prisms have to be incorporated into the spectacle lenses, contact lenses can offer no counterpart, as manufacturing this type of contact lens is virtually impossible.

Q: *Can I wear one contact lens if the other is lost or damaged or if one eye has conjunctivitis or a corneal abrasion or other injury?*
A: Yes. Wearing one contact lens will not harm the eyes; in

fact there are some circumstances where only one lens is ever worn (the X-Chrom lens for color-blind individuals, and the monocular lens for presbyopes and for some aphakes), as described in the chapter on special lenses. The eye wearing the lens will have good vision, and the other eye will have blurred vision. Many patients, however, cannot adjust to this type of vision and opt for eyeglass wear during this period.

CHAPTER TEN

THE FUTURE OF CONTACT LENSES

Any discussion of the future of contact lenses should begin with the human element—the eye doctor and the consumer. Forty years ago Theodore Obrig, a pioneer in the contact lens field, observed that "the fitting and prescribing of contact lenses is a complicated subject which requires knowledge in the fields of ophthalmology, anatomy, physiology, biochemistry, optics, psychology, and the specialist techniques of its particular fields." This is as true today as it will be in the future. It is not enough for the specialist to know about contact lenses: he must also be familiar with polymer chemistry, corneal physiology, oxygen transmission, the hydrodynamics of tear flow—and so on. More and more patients will demand better eye care and refuse to settle for less-than-optimal fitting, or inadequate information about what they can and cannot expect from their lenses. They will wisely demand premium care, and be willing to pay premium prices for it.

Contact lenses themselves are also improving, and the lenses available today will no doubt be replaced by even better lenses tomorrow. The ideal lens—one that can provide excellent vision and be worn round-the-clock without ever harming the eye—has not yet been developed. But the future looks rosy as the research continues.

Short-term developments will concentrate on improving the fit, comfort, vision, and oxygen permeability of the lenses we already have. Contact lenses will become a greater part of one's life with an increase in both full-time and part-time wearers. Though the big push will be behind soft, gas-permeable, and extended-wear lenses, it is unlikely that hard (PMMA) lenses will disappear completely. This material has performed so well over the decades that it will continue to be the lens of choice for many wearers for some time to come, although in modified form. Sophisticated research in polymer molecular structure—unhampered by the strict FDA regulations that shackle soft and gas-permeable lens research and development—may yield a lens that has a low wetting angle and improved gas permeability. Solving these problems would allow this old standby to compete favorably with other types of lenses.

Techniques for measuring corneas to achieve a better lens-cornea relationship are in the investigational stage. Eventually laboratories may be able to produce soft lenses as well as hard and gas-permeable lenses tailored to fit the individual cornea. Needless to say, individually produced lenses would reduce the problems of inadequate fit and poor vision.

If and when a reclassification of non-PMMA lenses comes about, new products will no longer need to go through the miles of red tape in order to gain approval from the FDA. It seems logical to conclude that we will see an increase in the number of innovative designs which will be less expensive to develop and market, and will also reach the eager consumer sooner and at a less costly investment. Just around the corner will be better bifocal lenses, better soft toric lenses to correct astigmatism, and extended-wear lenses for the astigmatic, the farsighted, and the presbyope.

All types of extended wear contacts will also be important in the future contact lens market. Heyer Schulte, a contact lens manufacturer, has predicted that by 1985 there will be at least six companies with extended-wear lenses on the market, and that 25 percent of all contact lens fittings and refittings will be for this type of lens. Although the gas-permeable materials silicone and cellulose acetate butyrate (CAB) show promise, it is generally agreed that soft lenses will remain the lens of choice for extended wear. Many practitioners feel that extended wear is *the* lens of the future, and the ideal lens—if one ever is developed—will be able to be worn continuously for many weeks, without the problem of deposit formation that plague this type of lens in its present form.

Extended wear has always been a dream for contact lens

manufacturers, doctors, and wearers, and some of the more imaginative predictions and experiments have centered around this highly desirable characteristic. A lens that was developed to be "glued" permanently to the eye was an eventual failure, but perhaps the disposable protein lenses now under development will succeed. A French firm, the Essilor Company, is experimenting with this type of extended-wear lens, which is made by a process that converts animal protein into a polymer hydrogel soft lens with a water content of 80 percent. They hope for a lens that is inexpensive enough to discard when it "wears out." Imagine a contact lens that requires no solutions and only one insertion and removal. You would buy a year's supply of such lenses, the price of which would approximate the cost of maintaining today's lenses. You simply remove the lens from its sterile packet, wear it until it needs to be discarded (probably from one to two months), and replace it with a new lens.

On the research drawing board is a concept that may be dubbed "instant contact lenses." This would involve the use of a special liquid plastic, chosen with the patient's prescription and cornea in mind. Once the correct viscosity plastic is determined, a carefully measured drop of the material will be placed on the cornea, where it will harden into a contact lens.

The various innovations previously discussed are what make the field of contact lenses so dynamic and exciting. Making predictions is dangerous in a field that sees new products arise with breathtaking—if not dizzying—regularity. The only thing that's perfectly clear is that the final chapter of the contact lens story has yet to be written.

CHAPTER ELEVEN

GLOSSARY

Accommodation. The adjustment that the eye's crystalline lens makes in order to focus on objects at various distances. The lens changes shape, becoming thicker or thinner through the action of the ciliary muscles (the tiny muscles within the eye).

Acuity. See VISUAL ACUITY.

Adaptation. The process by which the eyes gradually become accustomed to contact lens wear.

Anterior curve. The front curve of a contact lens.

Aphakia. Absence of the eye's normal crystalline lens. The lens is usually removed surgically because of cataract formation.

Astigmatism. A refractive error that is caused by unequal curvatures in the shape of the CORNEA; occasionally the curvature of the lens of the eye is at fault. Because of the irregularities the image does not focus at one point on the RETINA and is therefore blurred.

Bifocal. A lens that has two prescriptions—one for near and one for distance.

Binocular vision. The ability of both eyes to focus simultaneously on an object and fuse the two images into one.

Bullous keratopathy. A corneal abnormality in which blisters form on its front surface.

Cataract. A condition in which the crystalline lens of the eye becomes opaque, and vision becomes blurred.

Cleaning solution. A special solution formulated to clean the surface of a contact lens; it removes dirt, deposits, and harmful microorganisms that adhere to the lens during wear and handling.

Concave lens. A lens that has the power to cause light rays to spread out; it is thicker at the edge than at the center. This is also called a minus lens and is used to correct nearsightedness.

Comfort and conditioning solution. A special solution formulated to rewet, lubricate, clean, and cushion contact lenses while they are still in the eye.

Conjunctiva. The thin, clear tissue that covers the inside of the upper and lower eyelids and the SCLERA of the eye.

Contact lens. A tiny, thin, dome-shaped transparent disc that is usually made of a special type of plastic, but may also be made of silicone or a cellulose derivative. It rests on a thin layer of tears and is used to correct refractive errors of the eye.

Convex lens. A lens that has the power to bring together light rays; this lens is thicker at the center than at the edge. It is also called a plus lens, and is used to correct farsightedness, aphakia, and presbyopia.

Cornea. The transparent tissue that covers the IRIS and the PUPIL; also called the "window of the eye." The contact lens rests on the tear layer that covers the cornea.

Corneal lens. A contact lens that covers just the cornea of the eye.

Cosmetic lens. A contact lens that is colored and used to improve the appearance of a diseased or traumatized eye. It may also be used to highlight the eye or to change its color.

Crystalline lens. A clear elastic body suspended in the front part of the eyeball behind the IRIS. Its function is to bring the light rays into focus on the RETINA. *See* ACCOMMODATION.

Diopter. A unit of measure used to designate the refractive power of a lens.

Disinfecting/soaking/storing solution. A special solution used to store soft or gas-permeable contact lenses when not being worn; it kills harmful microorganisms chemically.

Disinfection unit. A heating unit used in the care of soft lenses that destroys harmful microorganisms by heat sterilization.

Dry eyes. Eyes that don't produce tears of sufficient quality or quantity. This condition may pose some problems for the contact lens wearer, especially if severe. In mild cases special lubricating drops ease the problem.

Edema. A swelling caused by excessive amounts of fluid in the body's tissues. Corneal edema occurs when contact lenses have been worn too long.

Enzyme tablets. Small tablets dissolved in distilled water to make a special solution that "digests" protein deposits on soft contact lenses, enhancing their wearing comfort and prolonging their life.

Extended-wear contact lenses. Newly approved contact lenses that can be worn safely for extended periods of time—days, weeks, even months in some cases—including while asleep.

Farsightedness. See HYPEROPIA.

Fenestrations. The tiny holes sometimes drilled in hard lenses in an effort to allow more tears and vital oxygen to reach the cornea, making the lenses more comfortable.

Fluorescein. A yellow solution that is instilled into the eye during an eye examination. The drops fluoresce, or shine, under a special blue light; this procedure is used to determine the presence of corneal abrasions, ulcers, and so on, and to assess the fit of a hard lens.

Gas-permeable contact lenses. The material of these lenses allows oxygen and carbon dioxide to pass through them directly from the air, so that the lenses can be worn longer and more comfortably. Gas-permeable lenses are made from silicone, or silicone and PMMA, or CAB (cellulose acetate butyrate).

Glaucoma. A disease of the eye in which the INTRAOCULAR pressure is increased to the point where the eye's function is impaired. The eye pressure is tested by a tonometer.

Halo effect. The term used to describe the rainbow-colored halo seen around lights at night when contact lenses are overworn.

Hard contact lenses. The first type of contact lens that was used widely; made of a comparatively inflexible plastic called PMMA (polymethylmethacrylate) similar to Plexiglas or Lucite.

Hyperopia (farsightedness). A refractive error of an eye which is shorter than normal, causing the light rays to focus behind the retina rather than exactly on it. The hyperope who suffers from this condition cannot see well close up, but can see images at a distance.

Hydrogel. The descriptive term sometimes given the plastics from which soft contact lenses are made; the literal meaning is "a gel that contains water."

Hydrophilic. Literally "water loving" plastics used to make soft contact lenses have a strong affinity for water. These lenses absorb water or tears; they may contain up to 80 percent water.

Hydrophobic. Literally "water hating" plastics that do not absorb water and from which hard contact lenses and gas permeable lenses are made.

Injection. A dilation of the blood vessels in the eye due to irritation. The resultant red eyes may be from contact lens overwear.

Intraocular. Within the eye.

Intraocular lenses. Small lenses that are implanted surgically, usually to take the place of the natural crystalline lens that has been removed due to CATARACT formation.

Iris. The colored part of the eye that regulates the amount of light entering the eye by dilation or constriction. As it does so, the center of the iris—the PUPIL—changes size.

Keratitis. Inflammation of the CORNEA; may be caused by contact lens wear.

Keratoconus. A condition in which the CORNEA becomes cone-shaped and thinner at the center.

Keratometer. An instument used during an eye examination to measure the curvatures of the CORNEA as an aid in fitting contact lenses.

Lacrimal. Pertaining to the tears or to the structures that produce or conduct the tears.

Limbus. The narrow boundary between the CORNEA and the SCLERA.

Millimeter. A metric unit of measurement: One inch equals 25.4 millimeters. Contact lenses are measured in millimeters and range from 6 to 16 mm in diameter and are as thin as .035 mm in thickness.

Minus lens. See CONCAVE LENS.

Monovision. A method used to correct PRESBYOPIA; in a variation of the monocle, one contact lens is used to correct one eye for close-up vision. If necessary, the other eye receives a contact lens that corrects for distance.

Myopia (nearsightedness). A refractive error of an eye which is longer than normal, causing the light rays to focus in front of the retina rather than directly on it. The myope who suffers from this condition cannot see well at a distance, but can see close up.

Nearsightedness. See MYOPIA.

Neovascularization. The development of new blood vessels in the eye; may be due to extended contact lens wear.

Ocular. Pertaining to the eye.

Ophthalmologist. A specially trained medical doctor who diagnoses and treats all eye diseases and disorders—through surgery, medications, and the prescribing and dispensing of contact lenses and eyeglasses.

Ophthalmology. The branch of medical science dealing with the anatomy, functions, and diseases of the eye.

Optician. A person who makes or sells eyeglasses and other optical instruments and who fills prescriptions for eyeglasses and fits eyeglass frames.

Optics. The branch of physical science that deals with the nature, properties, and origin of light.

Optometrist. A professional who can test eyes for visual defects and then prescribe and dispense glasses or contact lenses.

Optometry. The profession and applied science concerned with vision and nonmedical vision correction.

Overwear syndrome. The condition brought about by wearing contact lenses for too long a period of time. Because of a lack of oxygen, the cornea becomes swollen with excess fluid, the eye becomes red, irritated, and overly sensitive to light.

Peripheral vision. The area of sight surrounding the center of vision. This is interfered with during eyeglass wear; contact lenses not only do not block it, they correct it.

Phoroptor. An instrument used during an eye examination to conduct a subjective test that determines the degree of refractive error.

Photophobia. An abnormal sensitivity to light, causing discomfort; may be caused by contact lens wear.

Plus lens. See CONVEX LENS

Posterior curve. The back, or inside, curve of a contact lens.

Power. In OPTICS, the ability of a lens to correct a refractive error by bending light rays.

Presbyopia ("old eyes"). The reduction in the ability of the crystalline lens to accommodate. The presbyope who suffers from this condition requires reading glasses, BIFOCAL glasses, bifocal contact lenses, or a contact lens on one eye (monovision) in order to see close up.

Pupil. The black-appearing hole in the center of the IRIS through which light enters the eye.

Refraction. In OPTICS, the ability of the eye to bend the light so an image is formed on the RETINA. During an eye exam, the examiner determines the refractive error of the eye so that glasses or contact lenses can be prescribed to correct it.

Retina. Thin photochemical tissue in the back part of the eye upon which the light rays are focused.

Retinoscope. The instrument used during an eye examination to check objectively the accuracy of the results of the PHOROPTER.

Saline solution. A solution containing salt; in contact lens use, saline solution contains a concentration of salt similar to that of tears. Soft contact lenses are stored, heat-disinfected, and rinsed in sterile saline solution.

Sclera. The white part of the eye.

Scleral lens. A contact lens that covers the sclera in addition to the CORNEA.

Shirmer test. The part of the eye examination that measures tear production to help determine which type of contact lenses, if any, are best suited to the eyes.

Slit lamp. An instrument used during an eye examination to inspect the eyelids, CORNEA, IRIS, CRYSTALLINE LENS, and fluid of the eye.

Soaking and storage solution. A special solution in which hard contact lenses are kept when they are not being worn; it keeps them clean, hydrated, and aseptic.

Soft contact lenses. A type of contact lens intoduced in 1971 to the U.S. Made of a plastic called HEMA (hydroxyethelmethacrylate) or HEMA-like plastic, these lenses are soft and pliable and owe their comfort to their ability to absorb water.

Spectacle blur. This slight fuzziness of vision when glasses are worn may occur temporarily after the removal of contact lenses, especially if they have been worn a long time.

Tonometer. An instrument used during an eye exam to measure the INTRAOCULAR pressure of the fluid of the eye.

Toric contact lens. A special soft contact lens that corrects ASTIGMATISM.

Visual acuity. Acuteness or sharpness of vision. Normal visual acuity is usually expressed as 20/20.

Vitreous humor. The clear gelatinous substance that fills the eyeball and gives it its shape.

Wettability. The ability of a surface to accept water. A very wettable surface allows water to spread evenly and is desirable in a contact lens. Soft contact lenses are more wettable than hard contact lenses, which can be made more comfortable with the aid of a wetting solution.

Wetting solution. A solution used to "wet" the surface of a hard contact lens so that tears can spread evenly and readily over the surface, making the lens more comfortable to wear.

BIBLIOGRAPHY

Allansmith, Mathea R., M.D., et al. "Giant Papillary Conjunctivitis in Contact Lens Wearers." *American Journal of Ophthalmology,* May, 1977.

American National Standards Institute, Inc. Publication nos. Z80.4-1974 and Z80.6-1976.

Binder, Perry S., M.D., F.A.C.S. "The Extended Wear of Soft Contact Lenses." *J.C.E. Ophthalmology,* June, 1979.

———. "Clinical Evaluation of Continuous Wear Hydrophylic Lenses." *American Journal of Ophthalmology,* April, 1977.

Bitonte, J. L. "The Future of Flexible versus Rigid Lenses." *Symposium on the Flexible Lens.* St. Louis: The C. V. Mosby Co., 1972.

Blackhurst, Robert T., M.D. "New Flexible Silicone Contact Lens: A Thirteen Month Clinical Experience." *Contact and Intraocular Lens Medical Journal,* July–September, 1980.

Boyd, H. "Accelerated Wearing Schedule." *Contact Lens Medical Seminar.* Springfield, Ill.: Charles C, Thomas, Publisher, 1970.

Cavanagh, M. D., Ph.D., et al. "Extended Wear Hydrogel Lenses. Long-Term Effectiveness and Costs." *Ophthalmology,* September, 1980.

"Contact Lenses." [A two-part report.] *Consumer Reports.* May and June, 1980.

"Contact Lenses; Advances in Design, Fitting, Application." Selected Papers and Discussion from the 19th Annual Convention of The Society of Ophthalmology at Orlando, Florida. Edited by Joseph W. Soper, 1974. Symposium Specialists.

"Contact Lens Fitting." *Resident's Manual.* Department of Ophthalmology, Indiana University School of Medicine, 1981 (fourteenth edition).

Contact Lens Forum. Various issues from March, 1979 through June, 1981.

Duane, T. D., *Clinical Ophthalmology.* New York: Harper & Row, 1979.

Epstein, Gil, M.D., and Putterman, Allen M., M.D. "Acquired Blepharoptosis Secondary to Contact-Lens Wear." *American Journal of Ophthalmology,* May, 1981.

Fanti, Peter, O.D., and Holly, Frank J., Ph.D. "Silicone Contact Lens Wear III. Physiology of Poor Tolerance." *Contact Lens,* April–June, 1981.

Feldman, G. "Fitting Characteristics and Gas Permeability of Thin Hydrogel Lenses." *Contact Lens Journal,* December, 1976.

Freese, Arthur. *The Miracle of Vision.* New York: Harper & Row, 1977.

Garcia, G. E. "Continuous Wear of Gas Permeable Contact Lenses in Aphakia." *Contact and Intracocular Lens Medical Journal,* January, 1976.

Gasset, A. R., and Kaufman, H. E. *Soft Contact Lenses.* St. Louis: The C. V. Mosby Co., 1972.

Girard, L. J. "Corneal and Scleral Contact Lenses." *Proceedings of the International Congress.* St. Louis: The C. V. Mosby Co., 1967.

———. *Corneal Contact Lenses.* St. Louis: The C. V. Mosby Co., 1970.

Greene, James. "The ABC's of Contact Lenses." *FDA Consumer,* February, 1980.

Hales, Robert H., M.D., F.A.C.S. *Contact Lenses: A Clinical Approach to Fitting.* Baltimore: The Williams & Wilkins Company, 1978, 1980.

Hartstein, Jack, M.D. *Basics of Contact Lenses. A Manual Prepared for the Use of Graduates in Medicine.* San Francisco: American Academy of Ophthalmology, 1979.

Hollander, Harry, O.D. *Consumer's Guide to Contact Lenses.* New York: Sight Improvement Center, Inc.

Kaufman, H. E. "The Medical Use of Soft Contact Lenses." *Transactions.* American Academy of Ophthalmology and Otolaryngology, 75, 1971.

Kersley, H. Jonathan, and Kerr, Christopher. "Aphakic Extended Wear—One Solution to the Problems That Occur." *Contact Lens,* April–June, 1981.

"Lens Coatings Present a Problem for Extended Wear Contacts Patients." *Ophthalmology Times,* March, 1981.

Liebowitz, H. "Continuous Wear of Hydrophylic Contact Lenses." *Archives of Ophthalmology,* Vol. 89, 1971.

———, and Rosenthal, Terry. "Hydrophylic Contact Lenses in Corneal Disease. *Archives of Ophthalmology,* Vol. 85, February, 1971.

Lippman, Jay I., M.D., F.A.C.S. "Gas Permeable Contact Lenses: An Overview." *Contact Lens,* January–March, 1981.

Mandell, R. B. *Contact Lens Practice.* Springfield, Ill.: Charles C Thomas, Publisher, 1974.

Morrison, Robert J., O.D. *The Contact Lens Book.* Cornerstone Library, 1978.

New Orleans Academy of Ophthalmology. *Symposium on Contact Lenses.* St. Louis: The C. V. Mosby Co., 1973.

Pearlstone, A. D., M.D., and Blake, Robert F., O.D. "Parameters for Fitting Gas Permeable Lenses." *Contact and Intraocular Lens Medical Journal,* July–September, 1980.

Reynolds, Richard, M.D., and Sanders, Timothy L., O.D. *Contact Lenses.* Daly City, Calif.: Patient Information Library, 1981.

Roth, H. W., M.D., and Roth-Wittig, M., M.D. *Contact Lenses: A Handbook for Patients.* New York: Harper & Row, 1980.

"Several Types of Toric Soft Lenses Now Available for Patients with Astigmatism." *Ophthalmology Times,* May, 1981.

Simmons, Richard, M.D. *One Pair for a Lifetime.* Columbus, Ohio: Donald A. Keller Associates, 1979.

"Soft Lenses Successfully Manage a Variety of Corneal Conditions." *Ophthalmology Times,* April, 1981.

"Some Extended-Wear Contact Lens Problems Aided by Saline Eyewash." *Ophthalmology Times,* April, 1981.

Soper, J. W. *Contact Lenses, Advances in Design, Fitting and Application.* New York: Stratton International Medical Book Corporation, 1974.

Stein, H. A., moderator. "Symposium: How to Solve Flexible Lens Care Problems." *Contact Lens,* April–June, 1981.

———, H. A., and Slatt, P. J. *Fitting Guide for Hard and Soft Contact Lenses.* St. Louis: The C. V. Mosby Co., 1977.

Stranch, Lawrence A. W. "Relative Oxygen Permeability of Rigid Contact Lens Materials Related to Center Thickness: A Preliminary Report." *International Contact Lens Clinic,* January–February, 1978.

"Surfactant Cleaners Remove Adherent Lens Deposits." *Ophthalmology Times,* April, 1981.

Tripathi, Ramesh C., M.D., Ph.D, et al. "The Pathology of Soft Contact Lens Spoilage." *Ophthalmology,* May, 1980.

Williams, C. Edward, O.D. "New Design Concepts for Permeable Rigid Contact Lenses." *Journal of the American Optometric Association,* March, 1979.

INDEX

Dr. Spencer E. Sherman graduated cum laude from Princeton University, where he was elected to the scientific society, Sigma Xi. He received his M.D. degree from the Columbia College of Physicians and Surgeons. He is a Diplomate of the American Board of Ophthalmology and a Fellow of the American and International Colleges of Surgeons. He is an assistant clinical professor of ophthalmology at the Mount Sinai School of Medicine and an attending ophthalmic surgeon at the Manhattan Eye, Ear and Throat Hospital; Lenox Hill Hospital; Beth Israel Hospital; and North General Hospital; as well as a consultant for the United Nations Medical Department, the National Society for the Prevention of Blindness, and the Foundation of Learning Disabilities of Children. As a prominent authority in his field, Dr. Sherman has appeared on national television a number of times.

Nancy P. Bruning is the author of *The Cold Weather Catalog* (with Robert Levine), *Swimming for Total Fitness* (with Jane Katz), and *The Beach Book.* She has been wearing contact lenses for eighteen years.

Whether you're a newcomer to contact lenses or a longtime lens wearer, you will find Dr. Spencer Sherman's book an invaluable guide to the subject of life without glasses.

Individual chapters cover each of the latest and most advanced lens types currently on the market: hard; soft; gas permeable (including CAB lenses, which are made out of wood, cotton, vinegar, and natural gas); super-thin, extended-wear (recently approved); soft lenses to correct astigmatism; tinted soft lenses; soft and hard bifocals; and special lenses developed for such situations as color blindness. Dr. Sherman discusses the importance of the ophthalmologist's role, the pros and cons and characteristics of each lens type, which lens is the best and most appropriate for your life-style, and the scientific factors involved. There are well-illustrated instructions for each type of lens insertion, removal, and care, as well as detailed information on new cleaning solutions for allergic wearers. Also provided are aids in treating and correcting the most common and special problems arising from contact lens wear, suggestions for lens care while traveling and playing sports, tips for avoiding makeup hazards, methods for removing stubborn deposits from contacts, special blinking exercises, and more.

Illustrated with photographs and drawings

Spencer E. Sherman is a Diplomate of the American Board of Ophthalmology and a Fellow of the American and International Colleges of Surgeons. He is an assistant clinical professor at the Mount Sinai School of Medicine and an ophthalmologic surgeon at the Manhattan Eye, Ear and Throat, Lenox Hill, and Beth Israel hospitals, as well as a consultant to the United Nations Medical Department, the National Society for the Prevention of Blindness, and the Foundation for Learning Disabilities of Children.

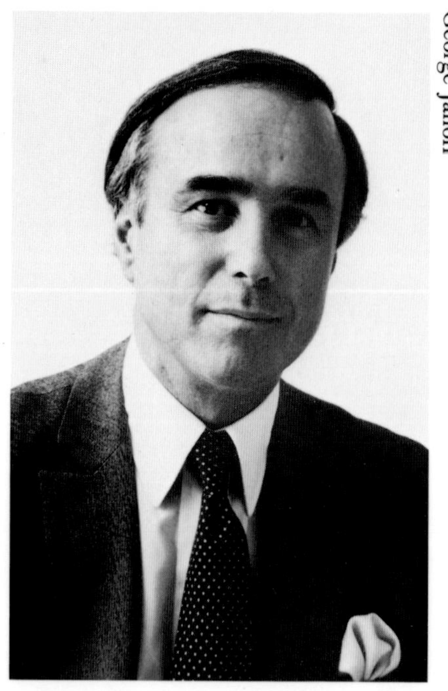
George Janoff

Nancy P. Bruning writes books and articles about health, beauty, and leisure. She has been wearing contact lenses for eighteen years.

Cover design by Jack Ribik
1082 Printed in U.S.A.

The Dial Press
1 Dag Hammarskjold Plaza
New York, New York 10017

ISBN: 0-385-2740